10-MINUTE
MAKE-UP

BORIS ENTRUP

10-MINUTE MAKE-UP

50 STEP-BY-STEP LOOKS FROM FRESH AND NATURAL TO CATWALK CHIC

BORIS ENTRUP

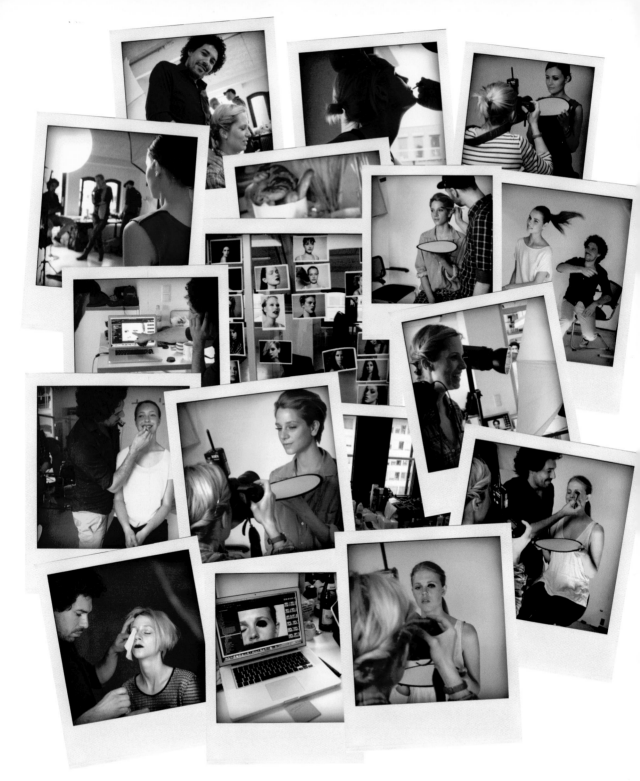

/CONTENTS

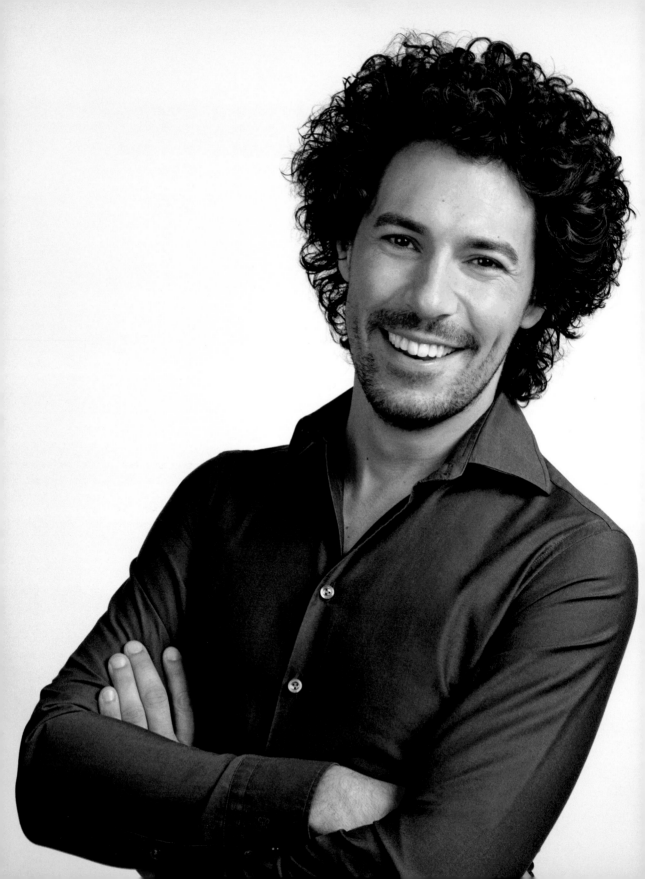

/FOREWORD

Go for it, experiment, stand in the limelight, and, above all, have fun!

I adore my work as a professional make-up artist and would love to pass on some of my own enthusiasm to you. "10-minute Make-up" doesn't just cover fabulous looks, it also provides countless make-up tips and tricks that can be used by every woman to create sensational effects in no time.

Make-up is wonderful because the transformation can be seen instantly, and the look you choose makes a very personal statement about you. Of course, there are trends, but there are no strict rules or absolute musts. Each new season brings new colours and textures to play with, and, the best thing is, you don't have to spend hours in front of the mirror.

In my daily work, I see which make-up styles are the most popular and which are less popular only because they are considered harder to achieve. But it would be a shame if you didn't try out smokey eyes or a dramatic eyeliner just because you didn't know the right techniques to use. Don't be afraid of colour. Dive in and experiment to discover what best suits your personality and your face.

The 50 looks presented here have been developed especially for this book. They are designed to enable you to create a look in ten minutes from a range of make-up styles. The looks are meant to inspire you, make you curious, and give you a push to discover your own personal make-up style. Step-by-step instructions illustrate the most important techniques and extra tips provide suggestions on every aspect of applying make-up. As I was putting together the various looks, I thought it was important to cover many different types of women and to make sure there was a look for every occasion – sometimes dignified and restrained, sometimes exciting and exaggerated. If you like a particular look but would rather set the focus on the eyes, not the lips, just vary the look and develop your own techniques and effects. Above all, have a lot of fun with make-up!

I hope my enthusiasm infects you and makes the world of make-up even larger, more colourful, more diverse, simpler, and more applicable to you. Have fun and be fabulously surprised!

Yours

BORIS ENTRUP

SKINCARE

Think skincare, skincare, skincare before and after applying make-up. Once every three to four weeks, treat your skin to a break by going without foundation, creams, or skin cleansers for a few days. This allows your skin's natural protective barrier to regenerate.

/1 TONER

Stimulating and refreshing, facial toner gently cleans your skin and makes your complexion look radiant all day. Facial toner is the ideal complement to gel or foam cleanser. Make sure it doesn't contain alcohol.

/2 PEELING MASK

A peeling mask contains microparticles that gently free your skin of dead skin cells and improve the look of your skin. Your skin will feel soft and look radiant. It is best to exfoliate once a week. You can also exfoliate with a hand-towel. To stimulate blood flow, simply rub the towel over the skin using small, circular, motions. This makes your cheeks glow instantly.

/3 GEL OR FOAM CLEANSER

A gel or foam cleanser frees your skin of dirt and make-up. It leaves your skin fresh-feeling, smooth-looking, and soft. Use gel or foam cleanser only at night. In the morning, all you need to do is wash your face with water and rub it with a hand towel. This means you start your day with a little bit of exfoliation.

/4 EYE CREAM

It doesn't matter if you use a gel, cream, or a roll-on. The delicate skin around your eyes needs extra care, mornings and evenings. An eye roll-on is a good starter moisturiser for young skin. Creams and gels often have richer skincare ingredients.

/5 COTTON WOOL PADS AND WET WIPES

Cosmetic cotton wool pads are used for applying skin toner and skin cleansers; wet wipes are perfect for removing make-up.

/6 CLEANSING MILK

Make-up must be removed, especially at night. It is very important to use a gentle, oil-free cleanser designed especially for the eyes. Cleansing milk gently removes make-up and dirt particles, and improves the hydration of the skin.

/7 FACE MASK

When skin is freshly cleaned, it is able to absorb many nutrients. Select a face mask to suit your skin type. Clay works best on oily skin and draws out impurities, and zinc calms irritated skin. If you have dry skin, apply a mask twice a week. For other skin types, it is enough to apply a mask once a week.

/8 COTTON BUDS

Cotton buds are perfect little helpers for correcting mistakes made when applying eyeshadow, mascara, or lipstick. They are also extremely useful for softening colour and blending.

/9 MOISTURISING CREAM

A hydrating cream is like a thirst-quenching drink for the skin. Always use moisturiser each day before applying foundation and let it work in. Ideally, choose a cream with a sun protection factor. Feel your skin after moisturising. It should feel smooth all over. Foundation will collect wherever your skin feels raw.

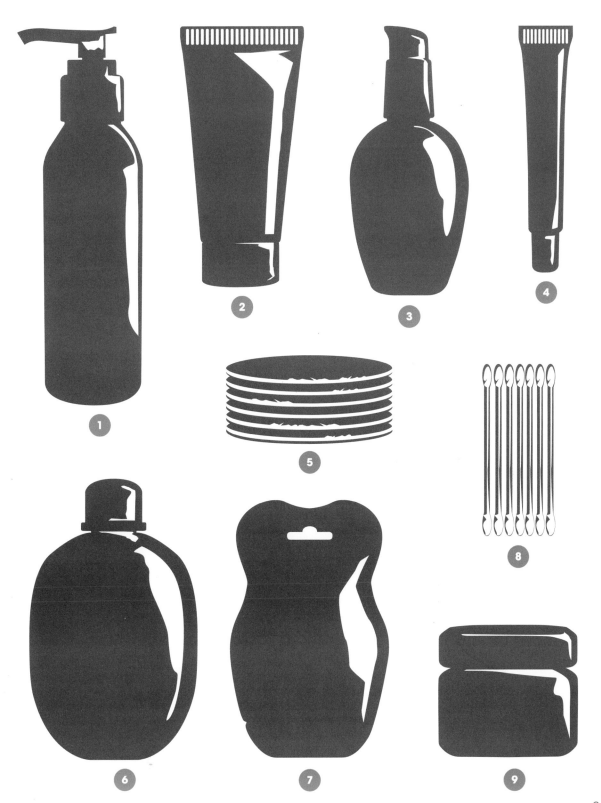

BRUSHES AND TOOLS

These 14 brushes and tools are just what you need to create the following 50 looks.

/1 POWDER BRUSH

Thick, soft, natural-bristle brushes are ideal. A soft tip ensures powder is perfectly and evenly applied to the nose and eye areas.

/2 BLUSHER BRUSH

The blusher brush is as wide as a cheekbone. Made of natural bristles, it is soft and has rounded corners.

/3 FOUNDATION BRUSH

The foundation brush has thick, rounded, synthetic bristles. Synthetic brushes are best for working with cream products, since their stiff bristles allow for precision work.

/4 CONCEALER BRUSH

The ends of the bristles of this brush should be half-rounded so you can easily reach the corners of the eyes and around the sides of the nose.

/5 EYESHADOW BRUSH

This soft, rounded brush is ideal for quick application of eyeshadow over the upper lid, or for blending.

/6 SMALL EYESHADOW BRUSH

With the help of this brush's narrow, rounded bristles you can do very accurate work. This brush is ideal for shading-in.

/7 ANGLED EYESHADOW BRUSH

This narrow brush has very short, angled bristles. It is ideal for drawing precise lines and accentuating eyebrows.

/8 EYELINER BRUSH

A narrower, pointier, angled brush with synthetic bristles, this tool is ideal for applying liquid or gel eyeliner.

/9 LIP BRUSH

The lip brush has long, firm, natural or synthetic bristles. The small, rounded tip lets you apply lipstick accurately.

/10 EYEBROW BRUSH

Well-brushed eyebrows are a must. An eyebrow brush with stiff bristles ensures the brows lie perfectly.

/11 PENCIL SHARPENER

Pencil eyeliners and lip liners should always be well sharpened. This is the only way you will be able to draw even and fine lines with them. It is really important that your sharpeners sharpen properly.

/12 TWEEZERS

A pair of slanted tweezers is the ideal tool for plucking out fine, uncooperative hairs. The tweezers' tip should be flat so you can grasp hold of even the tiniest of hairs.

/13 EYELASH CURLER

Only use an eyelash curler that has soft rubber pads so the eyelashes are treated gently. There are huge differences between eyelash curlers and here, too, you should opt for a high-quality product.

/14 SPOON

A perfect tool right from the kitchen! A spoon lets you apply mascara without small globs ending up on your eyelid. You can find out how to use a spoon when applying mascara on page 50.

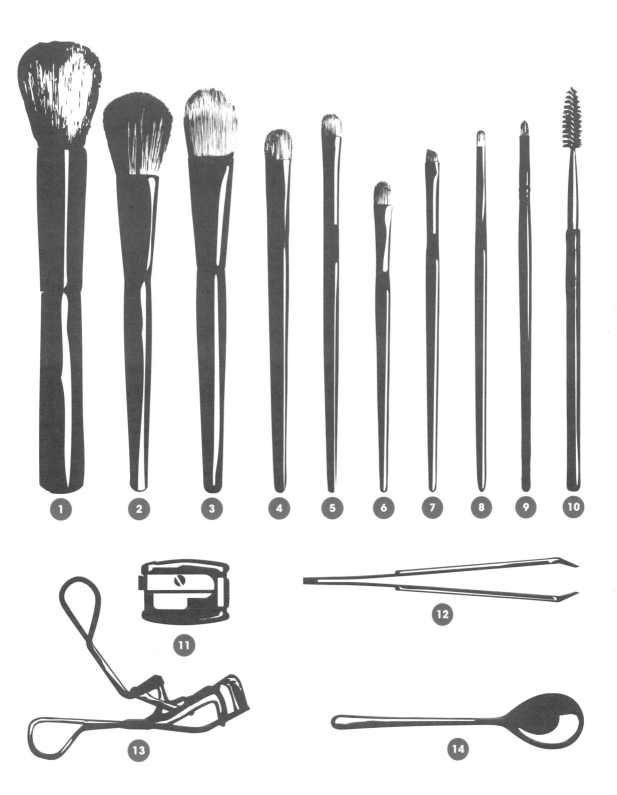

PRODUCTS

No more than four different products are needed to create most of the looks shown in this book. These nine make-up tools make a great basic tool kit.

/1 MASCARA

Whether it is used to create a natural or glamorous look, mascara is used in almost every make-up style. A curved mascara wand is well-suited for short eyelashes, since it reaches even the smallest and finest hairs. A comb-shaped mascara wand alllows for perfect separation of the eyelashes. Round, compact brushes make eyelashes look especially thick and voluminous. Don't wipe off the mascara wand on the edge of the mascara container, otherwise small clumps that have formed on the edge might end up in the mascara.

/2 PENCIL EYELINER

Pencil eyeliner comes in a variety of consistencies. You use it to draw soft, thick, easily removed lines on the lower and upper lash lines. Creating smokey eyes without a pencil eyeliner is unthinkable.

/3 OTHER EYELINER

No matter whether it comes in liquid or gel form, you can draw accurate lines with the fine tip of an eyeliner. After a bit of practice, working with eyeliner becomes easier. The best way to apply eyeliner is explained step-by-step on page 88.

/4 LIP LINER

Select a lip liner that matches your own lip colour. Use it to subtly reduce or enlarge the size of your lips, or correct tiny imperfections. Useful tips for drawing a perfect lip line are found on page 102.

/5 LIPSTICK

Lipstick can be dabbed on with a finger or applied precisely with a brush. The method used lets you vary the intensity of the colour.

/6 FOUNDATION

Foundation comes not just in liquid form, but also as powder or mousse. Various products offer different degrees of coverage, although this is not really necessary. Perfect make-up should look natural and not as though it has been painted on. Flaws are made to disappear, not with foundation, but with concealer. Apply foundation with your finger, a sponge, or a brush, and smooth in the edges carefully so the make-up blends in seamlessly and perfectly with your skin. It is best to use two tones that you can apply as needed. After all, the colour of your complexion changes even after a few hours in the sun.

/7 CONCEALER

Concealer is one of the most important make-up tools. With it, you can disguise imperfections, shadows, and dark rings under the eyes, and alter the face most strikingly. The perfect shade is a shade lighter than your natural skin colour.

/8 POWDER

Powder is used to set the foundation and give a matte finish to the skin. Transparent powder is best to set foundation. Coloured powder is used for shading.

/9 BLUSHER

By applying blusher, whether it comes as a cream, powder, or bronzer, you can give your face a vibrant look, and sculpt and contour your features. The choice of make-up style determines whether the blusher should be subtle or striking. Blusher tips for every type of face are found on page 34.

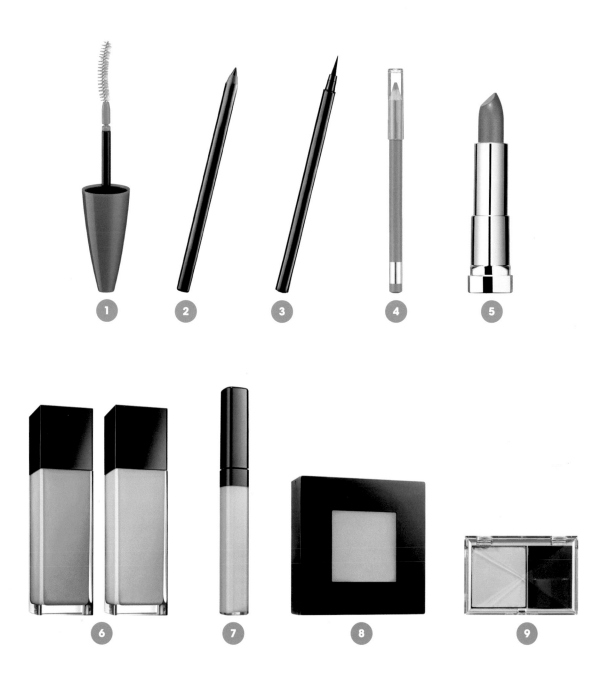

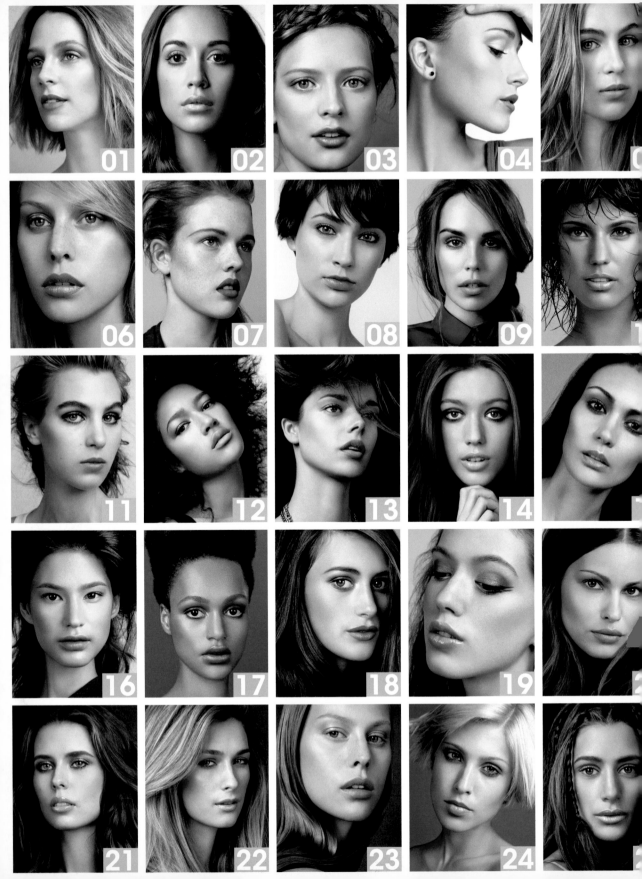

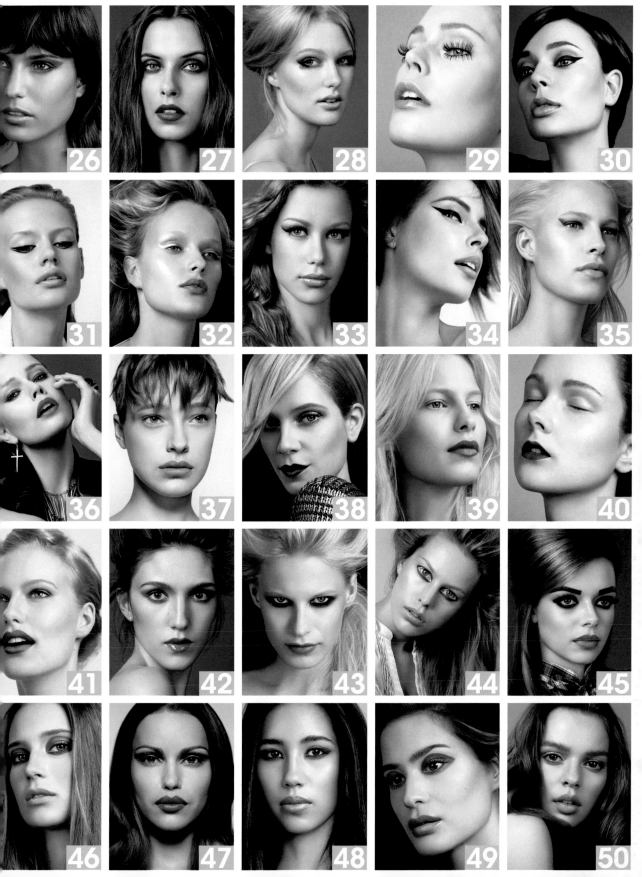

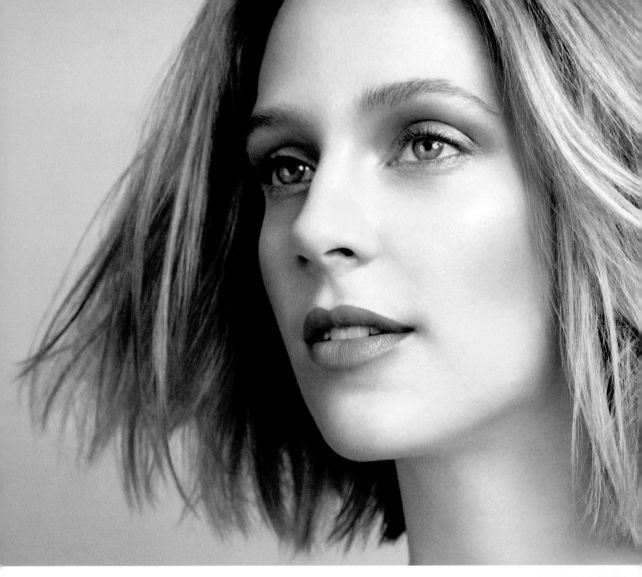

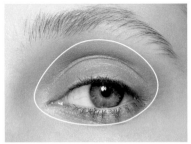

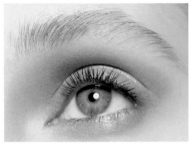

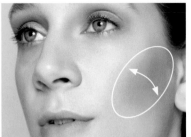

1. EYESHADOW

Using a rounded brush, apply slightly shimmery eyeshadow around the eye. Soften the edges to blend it in seamlessly with the skin.

2. MASCARA

Brush your eyelashes to make sure no eyeshadow particles are left on the lashes. Give the lashes a lift by curling them with an eyelash curler, then apply mascara.

3. BLUSHER

Apply blusher below the cheekbone and blend it out to all sides. Start by using just a little bit of blusher and only add more if you do not like the initial results.

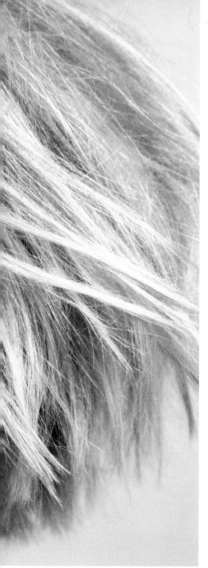

YOU WILL NEED:

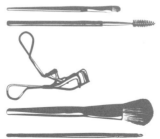

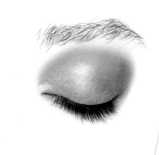

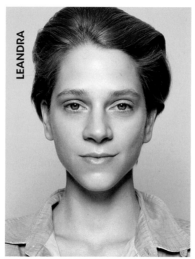

LEANDRA

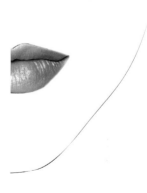

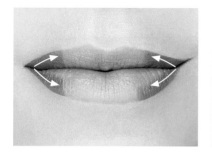

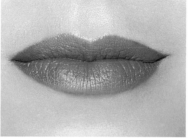

4. LIP LINER

First outline the exact shape of the corners of the lips. Small mistakes can be evened out in the second step.

5. LIPSTICK

When the outline is perfect, colour in the lips using a lip brush. To make the colour last longer, blot the lips, dust with powder, and reapply the lipstick.

/TIP: Dab on eyeshadow first, then use a brush to smooth it out. Since it is harder to get rid of too much eyeshadow than too little, it is best to start off with a small amount of eyeshadow, then add more as needed. If you end up with unwanted eyeshadow edges, blend them in with your finger.

17

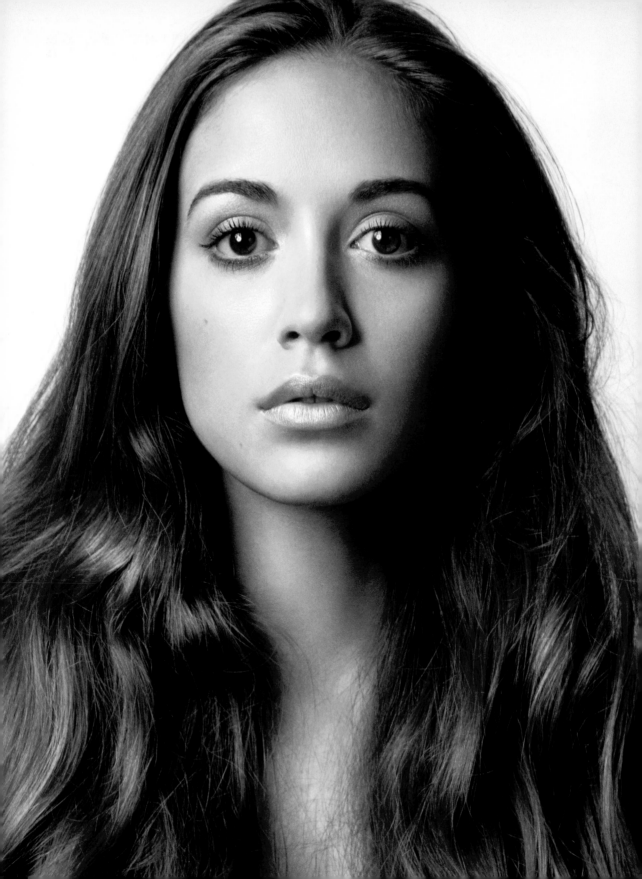

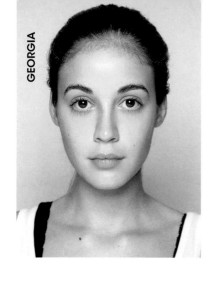

GEORGIA

YOU WILL NEED:

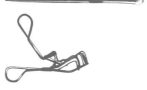

To get the best results when using mascara, make sure you use the right technique.

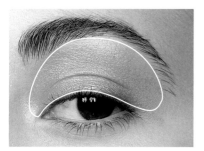

1. EYESHADOW

Apply bronze eyeshadow over the entire lid using a large brush. Then, blend in at the edges.

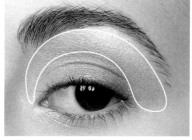

2. HIGHLIGHT

Apply light eyeshadow directly under the curve of the brow. Brush downward towards the inner and outer corners of the eyes. Make sure there is no skin showing between the two colours of eyeshadow.

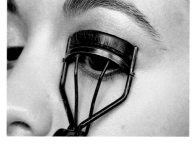

3. CURL

You must shape the lashes before applying mascara. Place the eyelash curler on the lash line and squeeze; then open the curler, and curl again halfway along the lash length.

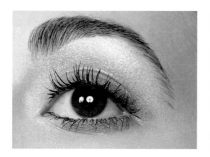

4. MASCARA

Using a mascara wand, apply a few layers of mascara along the lash line and only then apply it to the tips. This gives the lashes a great lift. Pay extra attention to the fine hairs at the corners of the eye.

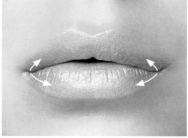

5. LIPSTICK

Pink lipstick with a pearly sheen goes perfectly with the shimmery eyelid highlights. Using just your finger, apply the lipstick, working from the outer corners to the centre of the lips.

/TIP: First, apply mascara to the really fine hairs at the inner and outer corners of the eye with the tip of the mascara wand. This step is very often omitted, although it makes a huge difference. You can reach even the tiniest hairs by lightly pulling up your eyelid with your finger. Then, apply three or four coats of mascara along the lash line. Next, apply mascara to the lash tips, and then to the whole lash length. You will be pleasantly surprised at the result.

BASIC TECHNIQUES: FOUNDATION

With foundation, you can sculpt the face beautifully by playing with the effects of light and shadow. As a rule, you need two shades of colour, one that matches your skin tone, and another that is deeper – a summer shade and a winter shade.

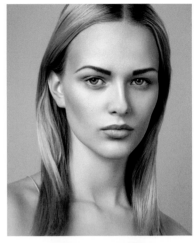

/FAIRER SKIN

YOU WILL NEED:

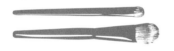

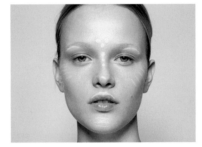

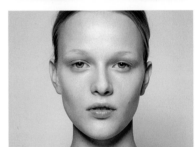

1. HIGHLIGHT
Using a concealer brush, apply the lighter shade of foundation to the forehead, bridge of the nose, chin, cheekbones, above the upper lip, and underneath the eyebrows.

2. SHADE
Gently work in the foundation so that the base colour blends seamlessly into the skin and your complexion looks smooth and even.

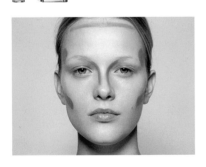

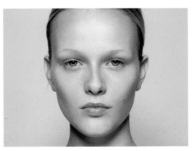

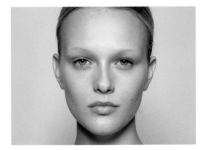

3. APPLY
The deeper shade of foundation is used to contour the face. Start at the eyebrows and work down to the top of the nostrils. Then apply foundation to the forehead, beneath the cheekbones, and to the temples.

4. SHADE
Next, carefully work in the foundation. This makes the forehead look shorter, the cheeks sculpted. Work from the centre of the bridge of the nose down to the sides.

5. PERFECTING
Make sure no edges are visible. The two shades must blend in perfectly with one another. This gives the face a perfect outline. Any asymmetry can be corrected afterwards.

Take your time when you are buying foundation.
Work the samples into your skin and see what they
look like after a few minutes.

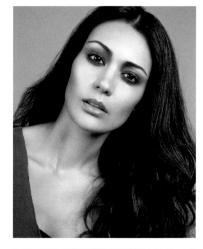

/DARKER SKIN

YOU WILL NEED:

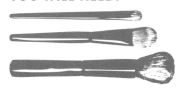

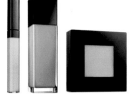

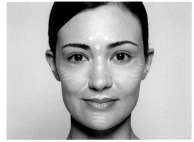

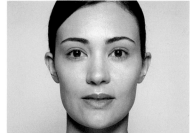

1. HIGHLIGHT

Apply the lighter foundation to the
inner corner of the eyes, beneath the
eyes, on the chin, forehead,
cheekbones, cupid's bow, and the
bridge of the nose.

2. SHADE

Now the eye looks more alert,
the nose narrower, and the lips
more defined. The shiny spots on
the forehead and chin create
great reflections.

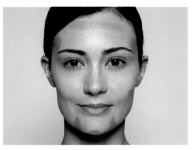

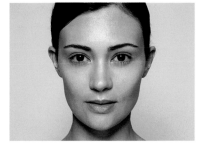

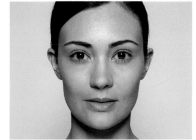

3. APPLY

Then use the deeper shade to
accentuate the nostrils, cheekbones,
and chin. Applying a deeper shade
to the forehead and temples makes
the temples appear narrower.

4. SHADE

Blend in the edges thoroughly,
working from the inside to the
outside. Check the result and, if
needed, apply a bit more foundation.

5. PERFECTING

So that the face looks well-balanced
and not mask-like, always blend in
the edges well so that they are
invisible. Set the make-up by dusting
it with translucent powder.

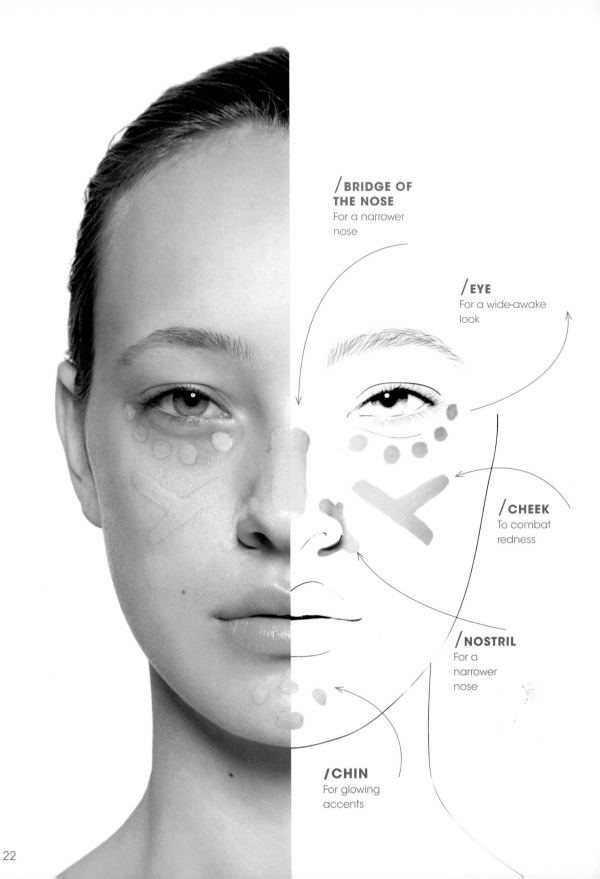

/ BRIDGE OF THE NOSE
For a narrower nose

/ EYE
For a wide-awake look

/ CHEEK
To combat redness

/ NOSTRIL
For a narrower nose

/ CHIN
For glowing accents

BASIC TECHNIQUES: CONCEALER

It is important to choose a concealer that is just the right shade for you. To find that shade, gently dab different shades onto the outer corner of your eye. Pick a shade that perfectly matches your own complexion.

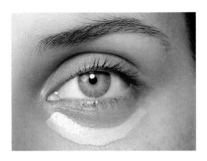

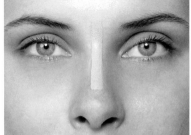

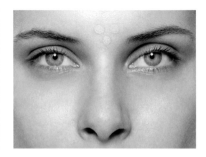

1. EYE
Apply concealer under the eyes, using your fingertips to lightly dab it on. Don't forget to apply concealer to the inner and outer corners of the eyes.

2. BRIDGE OF THE NOSE
Concealer doesn't just even things out; it also sculpts. Apply concealer to the bridge of the nose, but do not bring the line all the way down to the tip; this makes the nose look longer.

3. FOREHEAD
To open up the face and make it seem brighter, apply concealer below the centre of the forehead and blend it in gently.

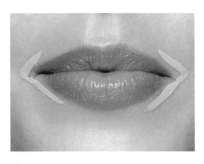

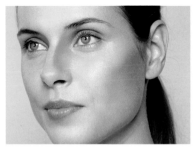

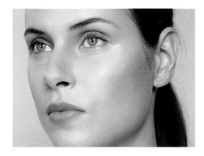

4. CORNERS OF THE LIPS
Apply concealer around the lips. Push it into the skin around the edges and all the way up to the cupid's bow. This defines the lips and makes them seem plumper.

5. CONTOURING
To give the face more contour, the nose and cheekbone are shaded-in with a darker colour of concealer.

6. APPLICATION
Now gently smooth in the concealer, working downwards. Do not rub too much, otherwise you will wipe off some of the colour.

03 \ SOFT ROMANCE

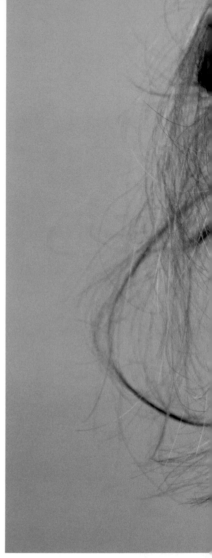

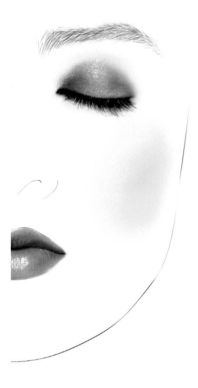

YOU WILL NEED:

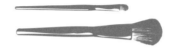

KAMILLE

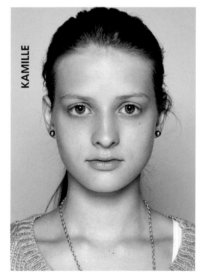

/ TIP: For this natural look, apply blusher sparingly and then thoroughly blend it in for a youthful look. Delicate pink shades are very well-suited to those with fair skin and blond or brown hair. In contrast, soft brown shades of blusher are ideal for those with dark skin and darker hair and eye colours.

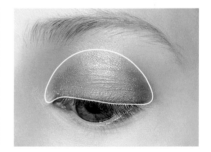

1. EYESHADOW

Apply eyeshadow with a large, rounded brush over the upper lid. When the eye is open, the colour should be just visible. The highest point of the eyeshadow should be above the pupil.

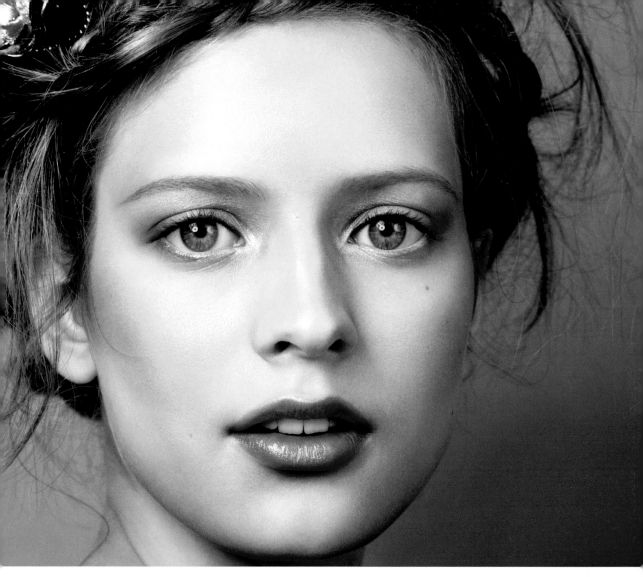

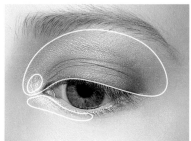

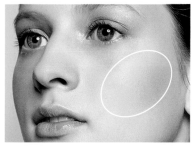

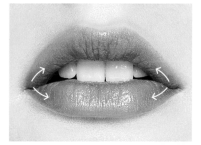

2. HIGHLIGHTS

Using a lighter shade of eyeshadow, highlight the inner corner of the eye. Apply eyeshadow over the entire lid, blending upwards to the brow line. Along the lower lash line, apply colour from the inner corner only as far as the pupil.

3. BLUSHER

Apply powder blusher to the centre of the cheekbone: blend it upwards to the hairline, then downward to blend in the edges. If there is a line, simply smooth it over with your finger.

4. LIPSTICK

For a natural look, choose a shade similar to your lip colour. To make the colour last longer, powder your lips after applying the lipstick, then apply another coat.

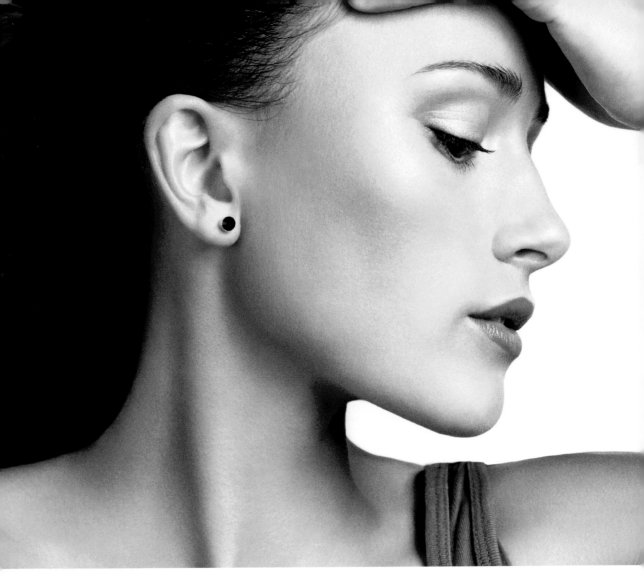

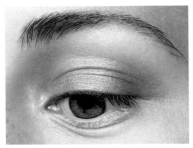

1. EYESHADOW

For a natural look, circle the eye with a light-brown eyeshadow that reflects the light. Blend in the edges. The highest point should lie above the centre of the eye.

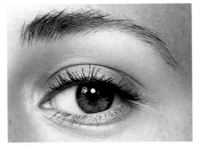

2. MASCARA

Take special care when applying mascara. When coated, the fine eyelashes at the inner and outer corners really open up the eyes.

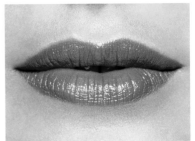

3. LIPS

Use a glossy brown lipstick. Shades of brown, no matter whether delicate or intense, flatter a suntanned complexion really well.

The copper tone in the blusher makes the complexion look fresher and more vibrant.

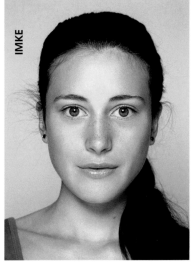

IMKE

YOU WILL NEED:

4. BLUSHER

Apply powder blusher to the centre of the cheekbone: smooth it upwards to the hairline, then downwards to blend in the edges.

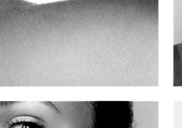

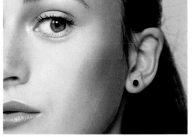

/**TIP:** A smaller brush is the most suitable to use when you are applying blusher as it lets you set the focal point precisely. Ideally, the brush should be about two and a half centimetres (one inch) in diameter. Warm shades of blusher such as apricot, coral, brown, or copper look best on yellower skin tones.

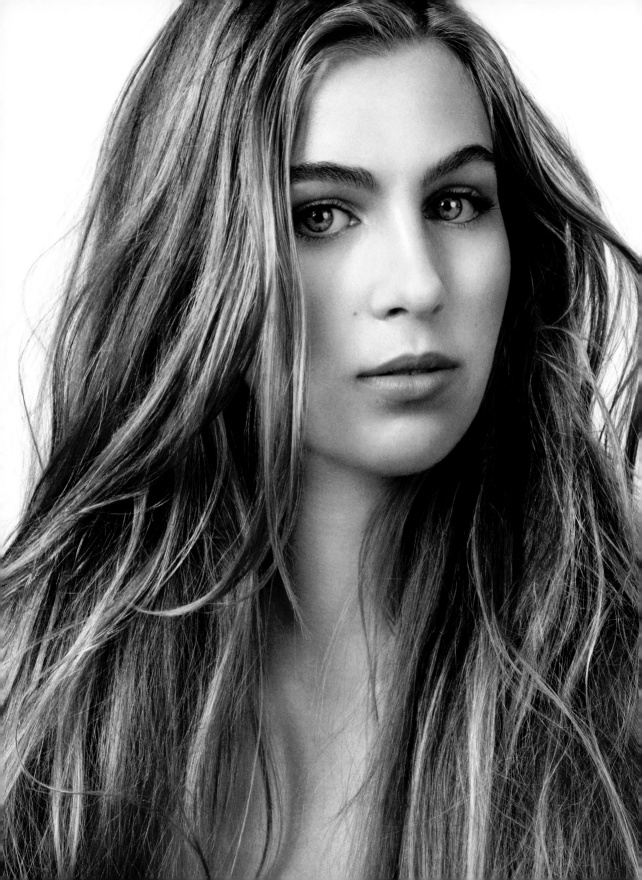

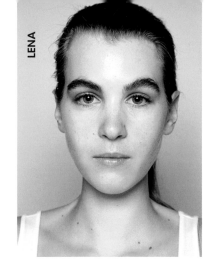

LENA

A brown shade of mascara is often better suited with a nude look since it gently emphasizes the eye.

/**TIP:** Don't fret about tiny imperfections! Instead of frantically concealing the dark rings under your eyes and blemishes, emphasize what you like best. This will draw attention to the right areas.

YOU WILL NEED:

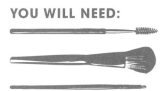

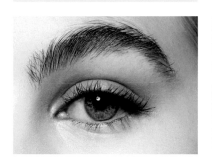

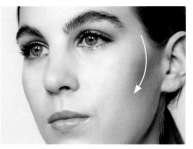

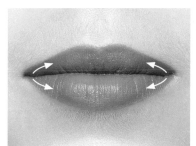

1. EYELASHES & EYEBROWS

Shape the eyebrows with a small eyebrow brush and apply a generous amount of mascara to the upper and lower lash lines.

2. BLUSHER

For this look, blusher is applied to the highest point of the cheekbone right beside the temple.

3. LIPS

Using a lip brush, apply a bit of lipstick to the lips. First draw the outline, working from the outer to the inner corners; then fill in the lips.

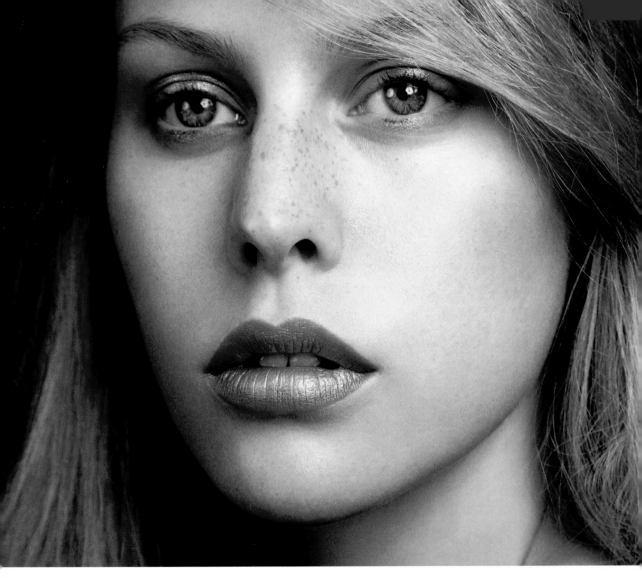

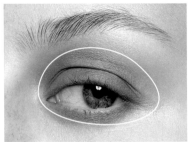

1. BASE COLOUR

Circle your eye with a light-brown, matte eyeshadow. You will get the best results when the colour almost seems to melt into the skin.

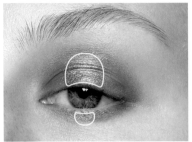

2. HIGHLIGHTS

Here, instead of a brush, use your finger to work in the colour. Dab on the eyeshadow above the pupil up to just beyond the eye crease. Then, dab it on the lower lash line below the pupil.

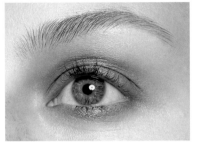

3. EYELASHES

Instead of using a mascara wand, put some mascara on your index finger and dab it on the eyelashes above and below the pupil.

Bronze is an all-purpose colour. It is a fabulous shade, as it suits most skin tones, whether it is used as an eyeshadow, a blusher, or on the lips.

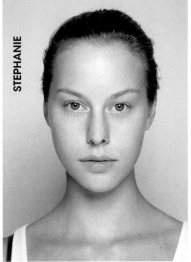

STEPHANIE

YOU WILL NEED:

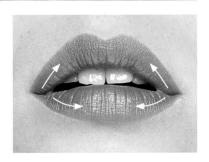

4. LIPSTICK

For a really lovely outline, apply lipstick with a brush. Work from the inner corners of the mouth to the centre, then fill in the lips.

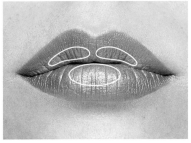

5. DAB ON

To mirror the shimmer above the eyes, open your mouth slightly and simply dab a bit of golden eyeshadow onto the centre of your lips.

/**TIP:** It is easy to work with your fingers. Often, you can better control the amount of colour you use. Also, your eyeshadow will last longer, since it is worked right into the skin. Soft shimmers, like those used for this look, can be created easily by dabbing on the make-up with your finger, which is a great tool for blending in!

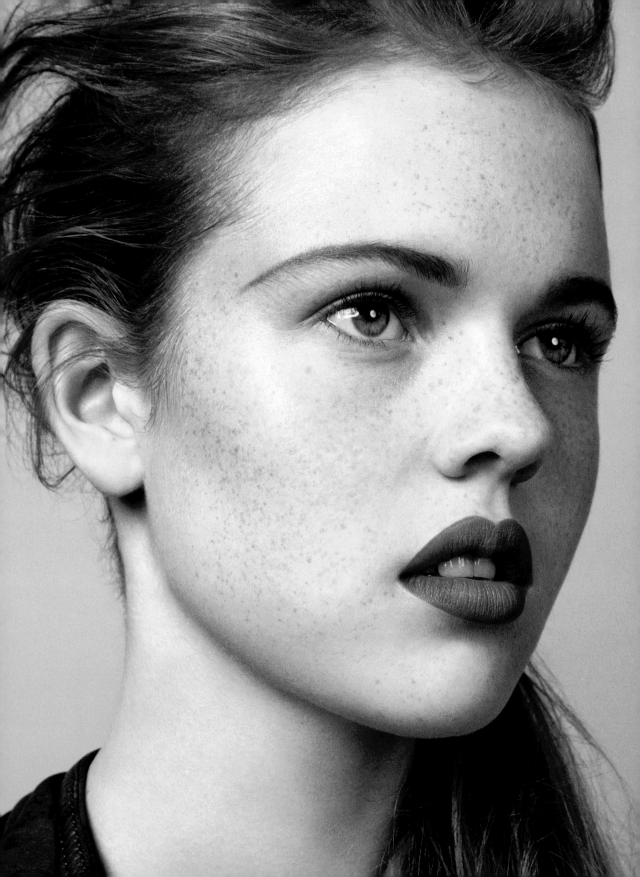

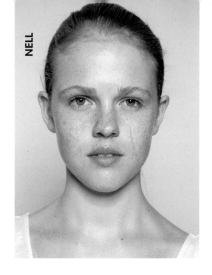

NELL

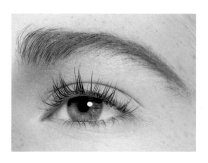

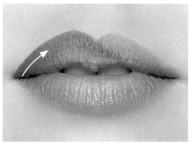

1. EYEBROWS

Using an eyebrow pencil, lightly trace the eyebrow line using fine strokes. Then brush the eyebrows well so that no lines are visible.

2 LIP LINER

A perfect cupid's bow is created with lip liner, working from the corners of the mouth to the centre in short strokes.

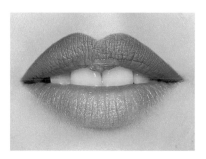

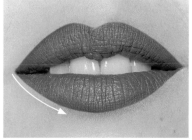

3. OUTLINE

Instead of painting the outline with lipstick, and for a long-lasting matte look, tighten your lips and carefully outline them with lip liner using short, solid lines.

4. FILL IN

Draw the outline of the bottom lip from the corners of the mouth to the centre. For an even line, rest your chin on your hand and hold the lip liner tip straight as you trace the lip line. Then fill in the lips.

/TIP: When the lips are the focus, the outline must be perfect. This is best done with concealer and a concealer brush. The concealer should match the skin tone perfectly; it should seem to melt into the skin. Place a bit of concealer on the back of your hand and pick it up on the brush. Then trace along the outside of your lip line and blend it in.

BASIC TECHNIQUES: BLUSHER

A touch of blusher in just the right place can make your face look fuller, narrower, fresher, cooler, or even wilder. If you have inadvertently applied too much blusher, you can easily cover the excess colour by using a bit of liquid foundation.

/SOFT

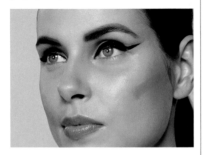

1. APPLY
Apply cream blusher or lipstick underneath the highest point of the cheekbone.

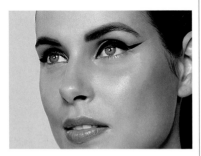

2. BLEND
Using your finger, blend in the blusher upwards to the temple. Smooth it in so that there are no hard edges and the resulting colour is as even as possible.

/DRAMATIC

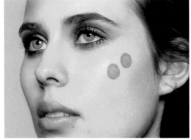

1. APPLY
For a dramatic look, apply blusher to the highest point of the cheekbone.

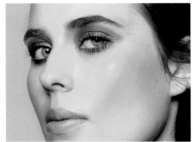

2. BLEND
Using your finger, blend in the blusher from the hairline to the corner of your mouth. To ensure soft edges, also smooth in the blusher upwards and downwards.

/COOL

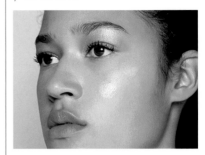

1. APPLY
Dab some light blusher on the highest point of the cheekbone and near the nostril.

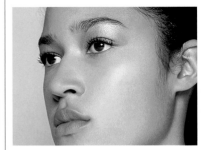

2. BLEND
For a cool and shimmery look, smooth the blusher downwards towards the nose and gently blend in the edges.

/WHERE TO APPLY BLUSHER

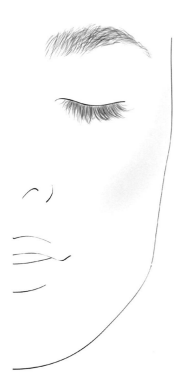

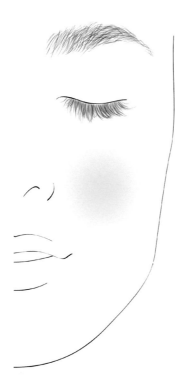

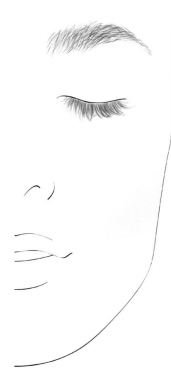

/V-SHAPED

To focus attention on the eyes, apply blusher to the temples and smooth it upwards above the brows in a v-shape and downwards to the cheekbones.

/FRESH AND LIVELY

To give your face a healthy glow, and look as though you have just stepped out of the yoga studio, smile and apply pink- or peach-coloured blusher directly to the apples of your cheeks.

/SCULPTED

For a sculpted look, apply blusher underneath the highest point of the cheekbones. Smooth it upwards and outwards into the hairline, then downwards.

BASIC TECHNIQUES: FACE SHAPES

With the right tricks, every face shape can be made to appear as perfect as possible. Whether your face is oval, triangular, round, or square, by following these tips, you will emphasize your best features.

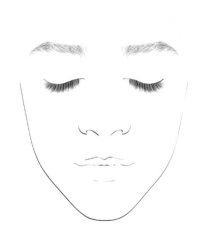
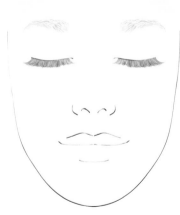
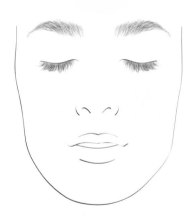

/HEART-SHAPED
NARROW CHIN

Characteristics of the heart-shaped face are wide-set eyes and a narrow chin. The face resembles an upside-down triangle. Lightly shade in the temples and cheeks with your blusher, creating a soft contour. This reduces the width of the heart-shaped face.

/OVAL
PERFECT SYMMETRY

It isn't necessary to correct the proportions when the face is oval. The blusher can be adjusted according to the look that is desired. Applying a bit of blusher above the temples along the hairline will serve to emphasize the proportions even more.

/LONG
RECTANGULAR

A long face is perceived as being too narrow and the proportions can seem unbalanced. Apply blusher to the apples of the cheeks, and shade in under the chin and directly on the hairline on the forehead. This makes the face seem wider and more oval.

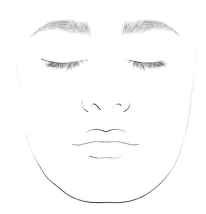

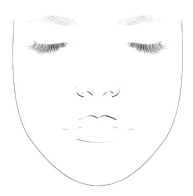

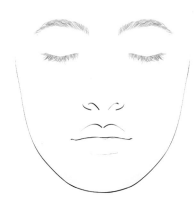

/SQUARE
BROAD FOREHEAD

A characteristic of a square-shaped face is that the widest parts of the face are at the temple and jaw. Project an imaginary oval on to the square face. Shade in everything that lies beyond the square.

/TRIANGULAR
PROMINENT CHEEKS

A triangular face has pronounced cheeks, which directs attention to the prominent chin. Shade in at the widest point of the cheekbones upwards to the ears. Repeat with the chin.

/ROUND
SWEET

The round face often appears flat, since it lacks defining contours. Broadly brush on a delicate colour of blusher right underneath and along the cheekbones. Shade in the jaw area and along the hairline. This creates a lovely sculpted effect.

08 \ PURE PENCIL EYELINER

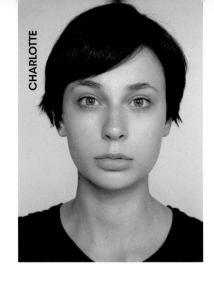

CHARLOTTE

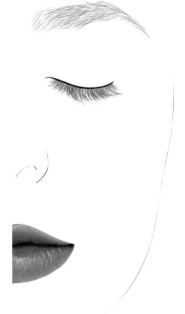

YOU WILL NEED:

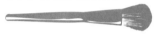

Most of us have a lipstick at home that we never use because the colour is too intense. Here is an opportunity to finally use it. First, apply lip balm to your lips. Then using a finger or brush, apply lipstick to the centre of the lips only. This creates a very subtle look.

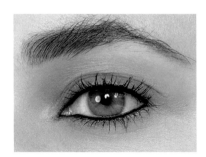

1. PENCIL EYELINER & MASCARA

Circle the inner rims with black pencil eyeliner. Also run the eyeliner along the upper lid at the lash line. This has a thickening effect. Then, apply mascara to the lashes.

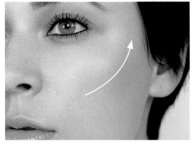

2. BLUSHER

Apply blusher to the cheekbone and smooth it upwards to the temple. So that you never apply too much blusher, first dust the blusher brush on the back of your hand.

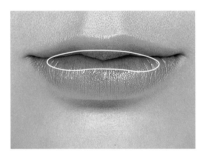

3. LIPSTICK

Apply lip balm to your lips. Using your finger, place a dab of red lipstick in the centre of your lips. The colour is the most intense where the lips meet.

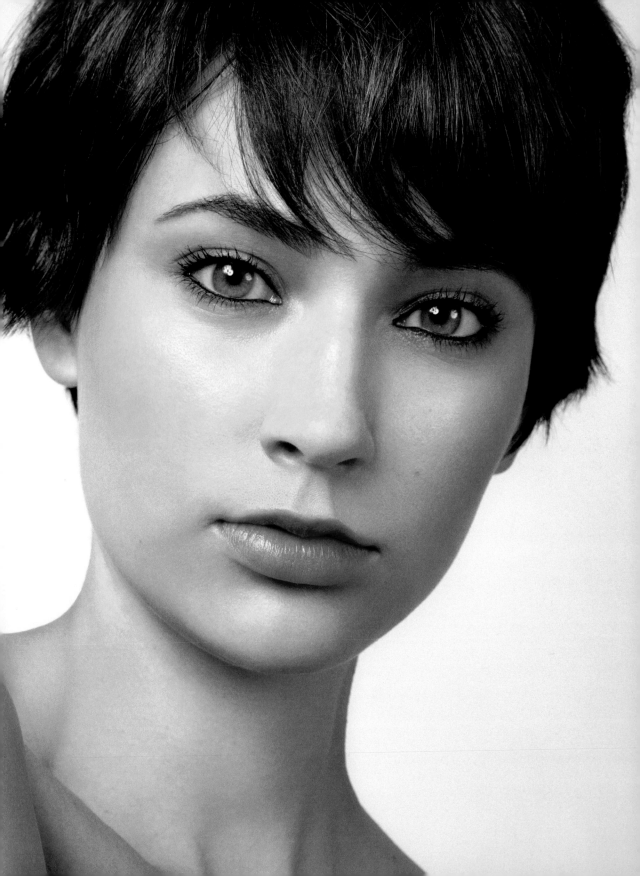

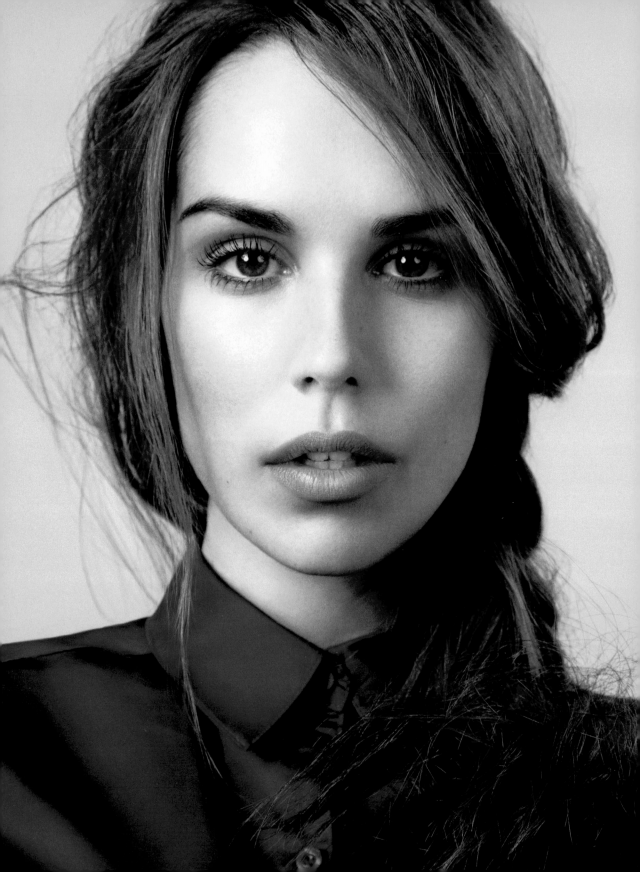

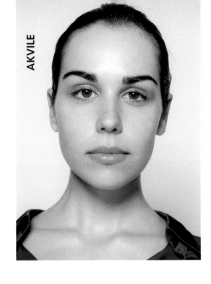

AKVILE

YOU WILL NEED:

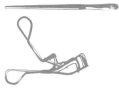

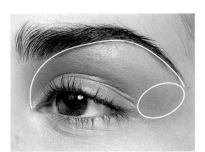

1. UPPER LID

Smooth on pink, cream eyeshadow from the inner corner of the eye up to just below the eyebrow. Using your finger, blend in the eyeshadow at the outer corner of the eye.

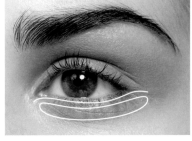

2. LOWER LID

Apply the eyeshadow along the lower lash line starting at the inner corner of the eye. Blend in the edges well.

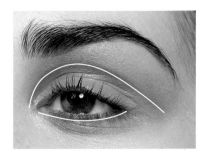

3. EYE CREASE

Extend the eye crease slightly upwards by drawing a line along and above the crease of your eyelid with a soft brown pencil eyeliner. Then draw a line along the lower lash line.

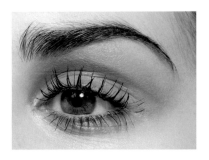

4. EYELASHES

Perfectly separated eyelashes are very easy to achieve. Curl your eyelashes, squeezing the eyelash curler very firmly. Then, apply several coats of mascara along the lower lash line, and finally, to the tips.

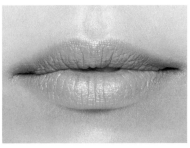

5. LIPS

Now, using a finger, dab cream-eyeshadow onto the lips.

/TIP: For this soft look, it is important to have a perfect complexion. Powder gives a wonderfully even complexion. It is best to use a small brush to apply it, so that the powder only ends up where it is supposed to be.

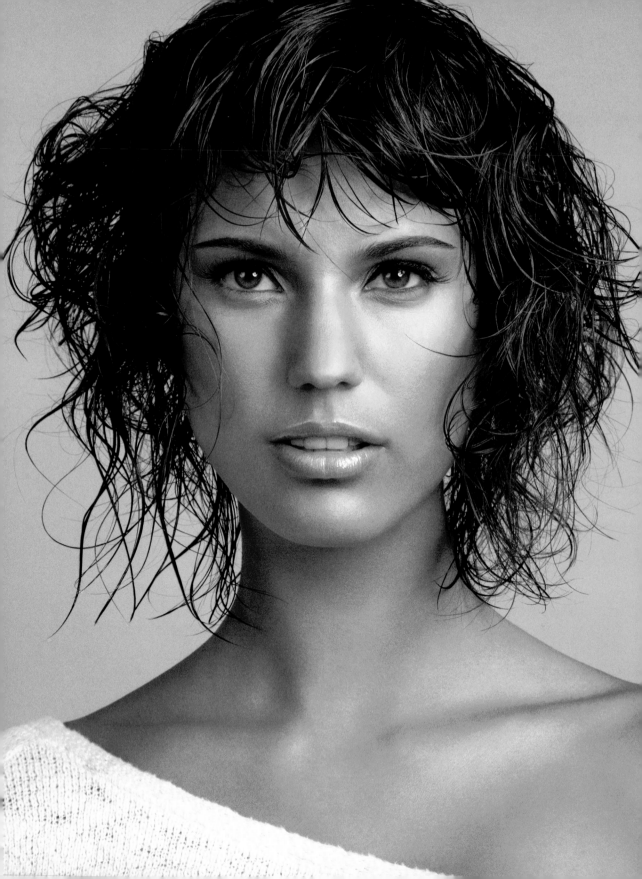

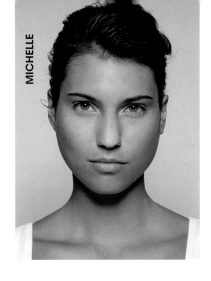

MICHELLE

This summer look suits everyone and can be created in no time. Apply several layers of mascara, line the eyes with liquid eyeliner, and apply a bit of glossy lipstick. Ready, set, go!

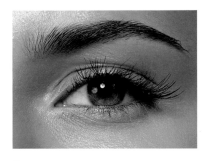

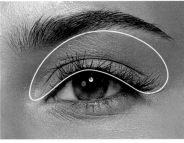

YOU WILL NEED:

1. MASCARA

Place the eyelash curler right on the lash line and squeeze firmly. Apply several layers of mascara along the lash line and then on the tips.

2. EYESHADOW

Apply brown eyeshadow over the upper lid and above the eye crease all the way up to the brow. Make sure the edges are blended in well.

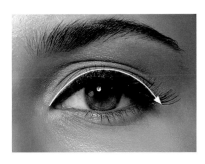

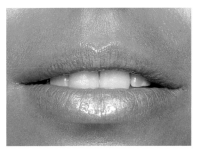

/**TIP:** Perfect skin hardly needs any foundation. Concealer is all you need, particularly when your face is tanned. Just apply concealer selectively to any dark shadows, and work it into the skin.

3. EYELINER

So that the eye appears larger and the eyelashes thicker, apply liquid eyeliner at the upper inner corner of the eye and stop at the outer corner.

4. LIPSTICK

To finish, apply a bit of glossy lipstick to the lips. The summer look is ready.

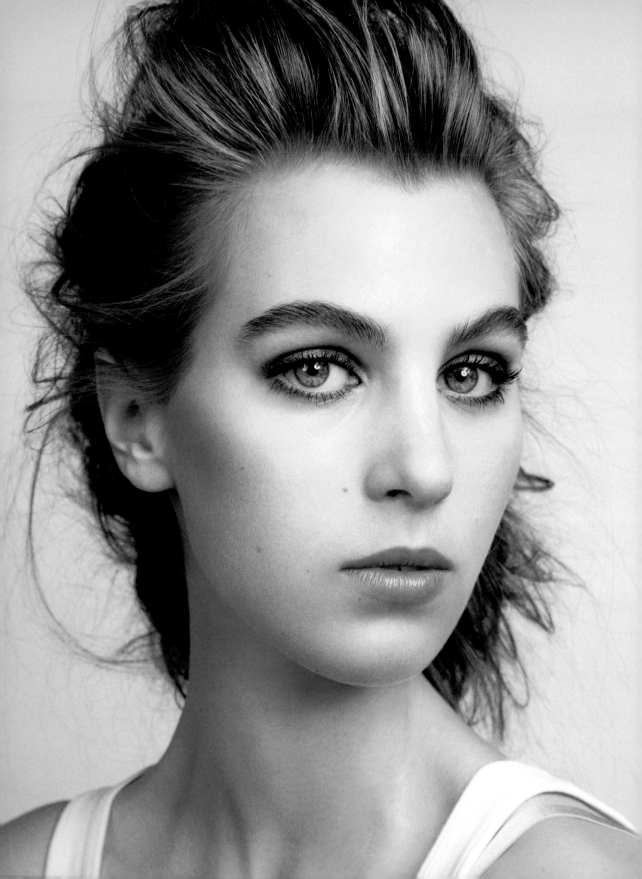

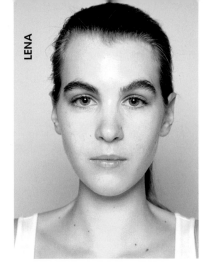

LENA

SWEET GREY /11

To apply eyeshadow evenly, work from the inner corner of the eye to the outer corner and then back again. This ensures the eyeshadow colour has the same intensity all over the lid.

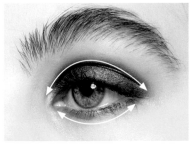
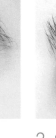

1. EYESHADOW

Circle your eye with grey eyeshadow. Work from the inner corner to the outer corner and back again on both the upper mobile eyelid and lower lash line.

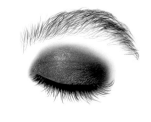

2. MASCARA

Shape the eyebrows with a small brow brush. Apply several layers of mascara to the upper and lower lashes.

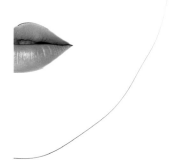

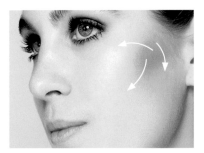

3. BLUSHER

Apply blusher to the upper cheekbone and smooth it out to all sides. This gives the cheeks a very natural-looking glow that makes for a radiant look.

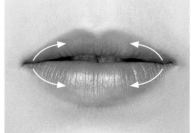

4. LIPSTICK

Working from the corner of your lips to the centre, apply a delicate pink shade of lipstick. Blot with a tissue, dust with powder, and reapply the lipstick. This makes the lipstick last longer.

YOU WILL NEED:

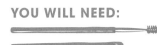

12 \ DUSTY LILAC

YOU WILL NEED:

LOVELYN

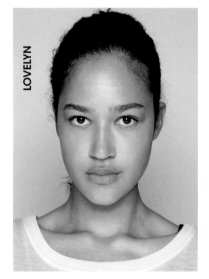

/**TIP:** Many products can be used for purposes other than that for which they were intended. For example, you can also use eyeshadow on your lips when there is no lipstick to hand – the colour is fabulous, and it's handy when time is short. To create a lip look like the one shown here, all you have to do is apply eyeshadow over lip balm.

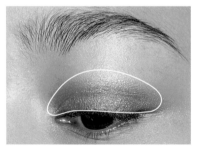

1. EYESHADOW
Using a rounded brush, apply shimmery-violet eyeshadow over the mobile lid.

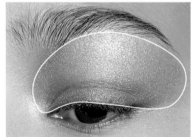

2. HIGHLIGHT
Using a larger brush, layer on a lighter shade of eyeshadow, blending the colour upwards to the brow line.

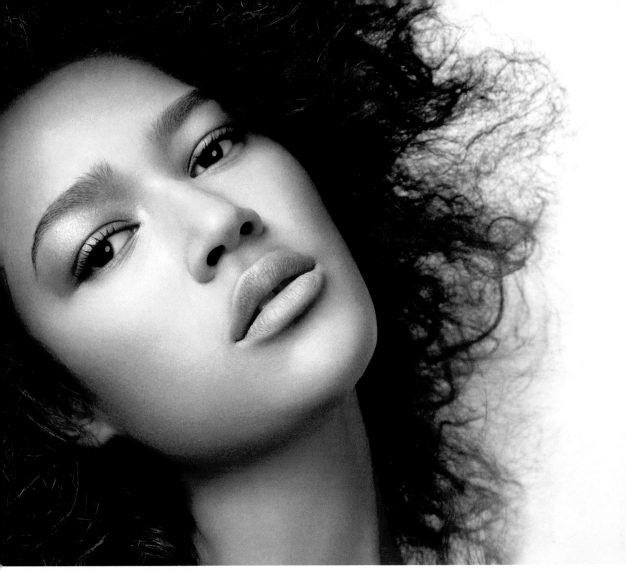

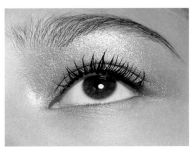

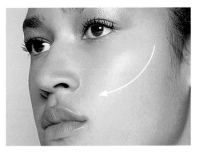

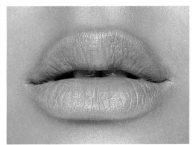

3. MASCARA
Carefully apply mascara to the top lashes. Make sure the mascara is also applied to the fine inner and outer eyelashes.

4. BLUSHER
Dab cream blusher that has a silvery sheen on the highest point of the cheekbone and near the nostril, then blend it in.

5. LIPS
For matte, understated lips, apply lip balm and lightly dab violet eyeshadow on the lips.

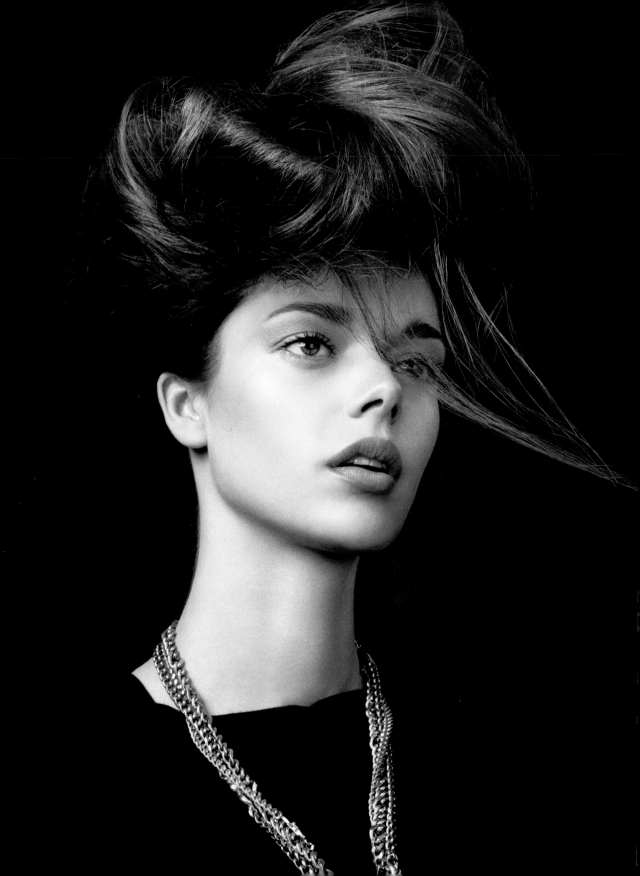

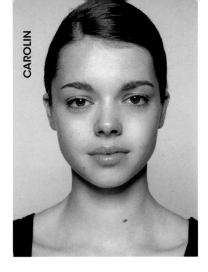

You can take the shimmer out of lipstick in an instant. After you have covered your lips with lipstick, set it with a dusting of translucent powder.

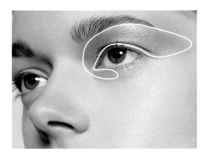

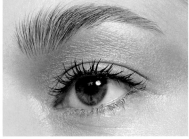

YOU WILL NEED:

1. EYESHADOW

Eyeshadow doesn't have to stop at the outer corner of the eye. Here, gold eyeshadow is applied to the inner corner of the eye, the upper lid, and then upwards to the temple.

2. MASCARA

Concentrate on the lash line first when applying mascara. Then apply mascara to the lash tips. This gives the lashes a great sweep, and they won't clump together.

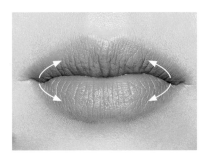

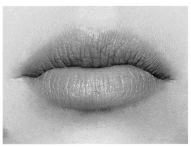

3. LIPSTICK

Here, a light coral lipstick is used. It is similar to the natural lip colour and results in evenly coloured lips.

4. POWDER

For a matte, subtle lip look, lightly dust the lipstick with powder after application.

/TIP: How can you apply eyeshadow without having some of it land beneath your eyes? It's quite simple. First, knock off any excess powder from the eyeshadow brush. Then, use the back of your hand to see how much colour is left on the brush. If a bit of eyeshadow does go astray after all, clean it off with a cotton bud and a bit of moisturiser.

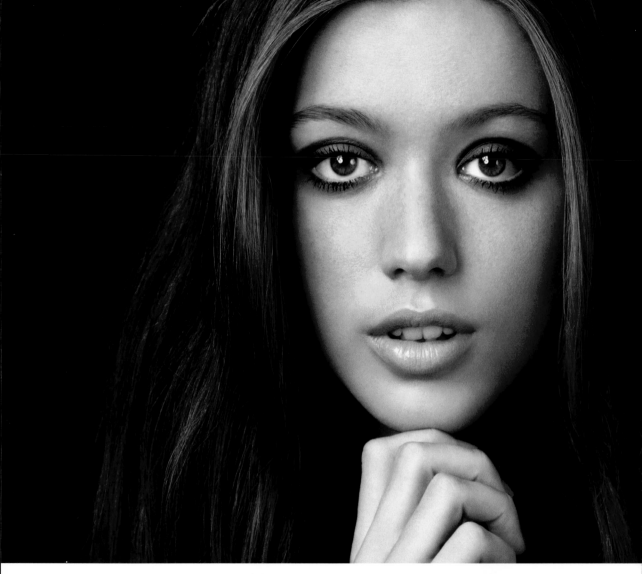

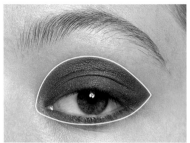

1. CIRCLE

Using a lovely, deep-lilac eyeshadow, circle your eyes in an almond shape. Start with a large brush, then use a narrow, rounded brush to follow the eye contour and define the shape.

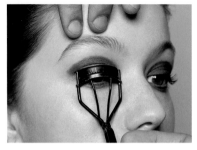

2. CURLER

Shape your eyelashes before applying mascara. Place the eyelash curler on the upper lash line and squeeze firmly.

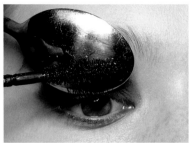

3. MASCARA

So that no mascara splotches end up on the eyeshadow, take a teaspoon and place it on the upper lid. Apply lots of mascara to the lashes over the back of the spoon.

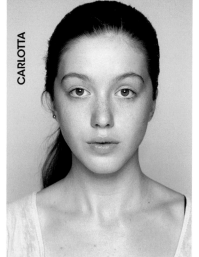

CARLOTTA

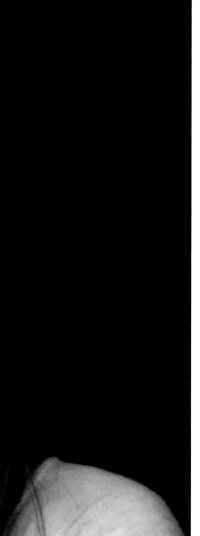

/**TIP:** Complementary colours are just the thing to make your eyes sparkle. To emphasize warm eye colours, use a cool tone and vice versa. For example, if you have blue eyes, pick a bronze tone. To make grey eyes stand out, use a warm, green tone. For brown eyes, a cool, lilac tone works very well. You absolutely must try this out and you will see how the colour of your eyes is intensified.

YOU WILL NEED:

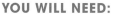
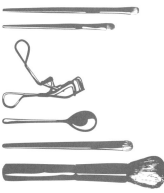

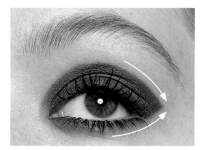

4. CONCEALER

To get the perfect outline, correct any imperfections with concealer. Just dab a bit on the back of your hand, pick it up with a brush, and trace along the eyeshadow outline.

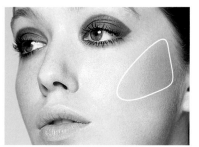

5. BLUSHER

For a fresh look, apply powder blusher above the cheekbone and blend in upwards to the temple. Always rotate the brush on the back of your hand first so that you never apply too much blusher.

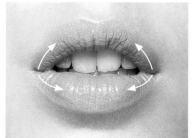

6. LIPSTICK

Since the focus is on the eyes, the lips are kept understated. Just apply a bit of pink lipstick, dust with powder, and reapply the lipstick. This makes the lipstick last longer.

15 \ CHOCOLATE EYES

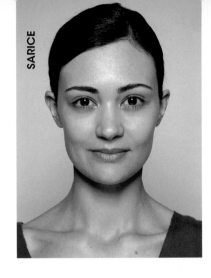

YOU WILL NEED:

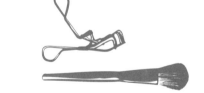

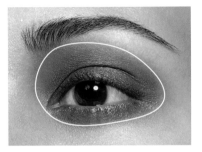

1. EYESHADOW
Using a rounded brush, circle your eye with chocolate-brown eyeshadow powder. Using a larger brush, soften the edges.

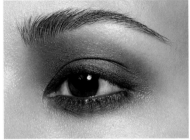

2. PENCIL EYELINER
For even more expressive eyes, outline the eyes with a pencil eyeliner that matches the eyeshadow. Don't forget the inner corners. Then, brush eyeshadow over the eyeliner to set it.

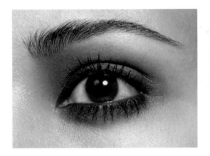

3. MASCARA
To finish off this sensuous eye make-up, curl your eyelashes to give them a lift and then apply lots of mascara.

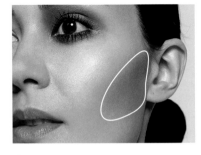

4. OUTLINE
Use dark face powder to sculpt the face. Shade in the area below the cheekbone and upwards to the temple.

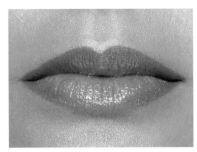

5. GLOSS
Just use light nude gloss to emphasize your natural lip colour.

/TIP: There are countless ways of emphasizing brown eyes. Tone-on-tone makes brown eyes look sensuous. Colours such as lilac, green, and grey make eyes really stand out. Cool colours, in particular, really accentuate brown eyes – just try it out!

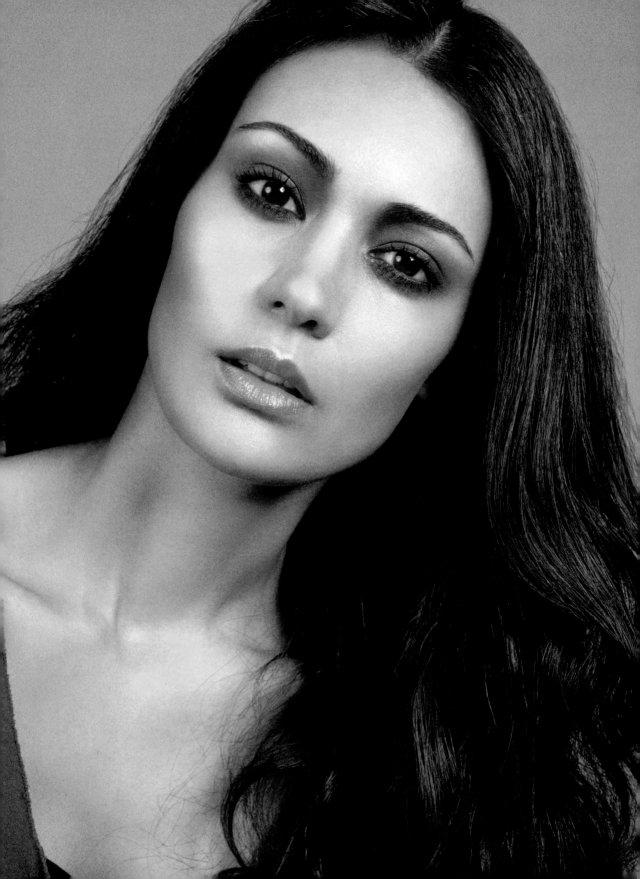

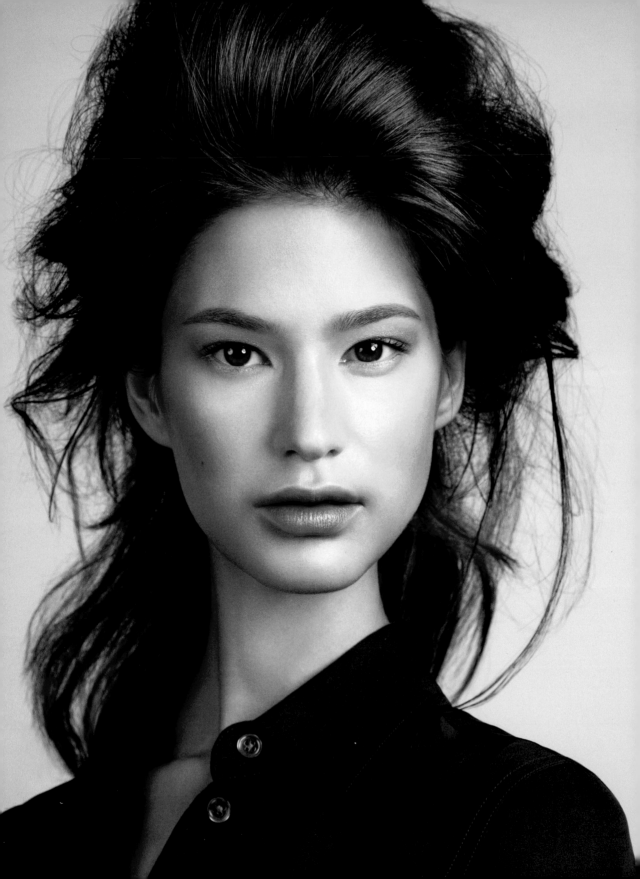

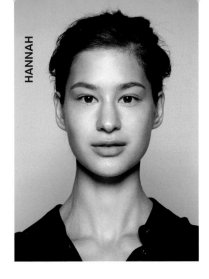

YOU WILL NEED:

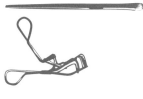

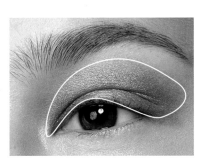

1. EYESHADOW

Apply eyeshadow over the entire upper lid. The highest point should be above the outer side of the pupil.

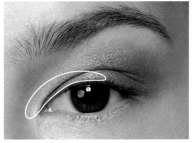

2. HIGHLIGHT

Use white eyeshadow to highlight the inner corner of the eye. Blend in the highlighter to the centre of the pupil.

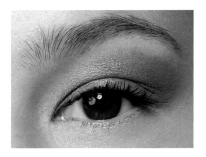

3. MASCARA

Curl the eyelashes with an eyelash curler and apply mascara thickly to the upper lashes.

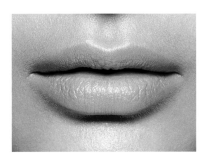

4. SOFTEN

The lips can be softened to understate them. To create this effect, apply a bit of lip balm to the lips, then dab on a bit of foundation.

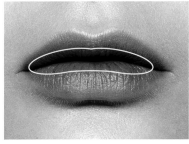

5. LIPSTICK

Using your fingertip, dab a bit of intensely coloured lipstick on the centre of the lips.

/**TIP:** The highest point of the eyeshadow doesn't always have to be above the pupil. If you have narrow eyes, the highest point can be set above the outer side of the pupil. This makes the eyes look almond-shaped.

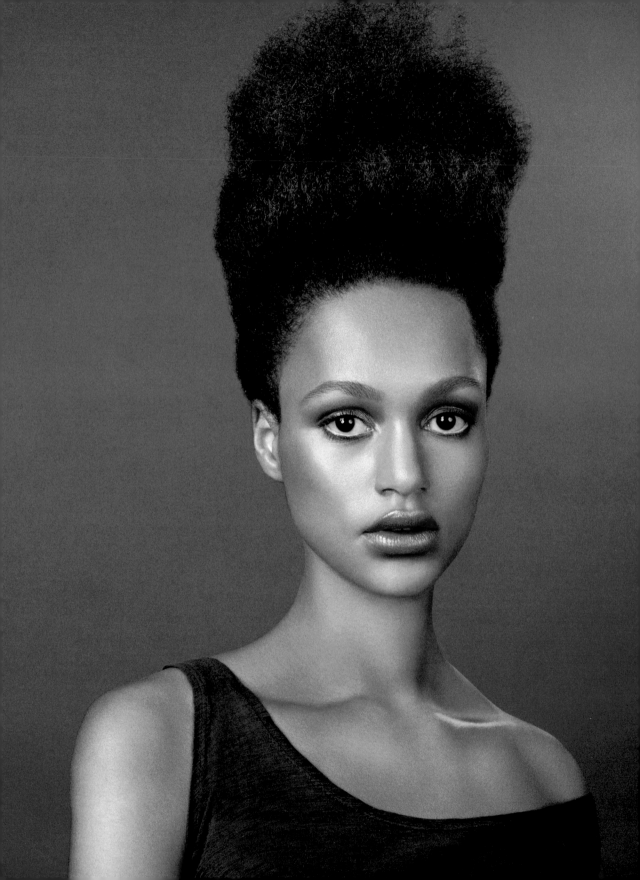

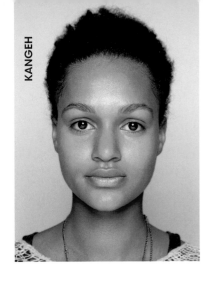

KANGEH

YOU WILL NEED:

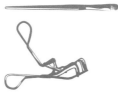

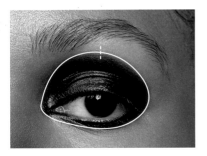

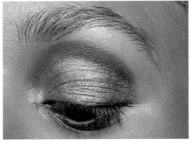

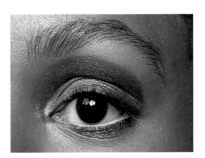

1. PENCIL EYELINER
Circle your eye with pencil eyeliner. The highest point should lie above the centre of the pupil. Make the eyes look larger by extending the eyeliner from the inner corner of the eye to beyond the outer corner.

2. EYESHADOW
Apply a metallic-colour eyeshadow with a rounded brush right on top of the pencil eyeliner. This gives the colour an entirely new intensity.

3. WHITE PENCIL EYELINER
To make the eye colour pop out, line the inner rim with white pencil eyeliner.

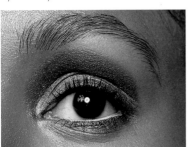

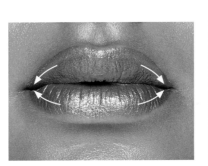

4. MASCARA
Curl the eyelashes with an eyelash curler. Then generously apply mascara to the upper and lower lashes. First apply mascara to the lash line, then to the tips of the lashes.

5. GLOSS
Bronze gloss echoes the shimmer around the eyes perfectly. Just dab it on the centre of the lips and gently smooth it outwards over the lips.

/**TIP:** Eyeshadow lasts longest and has the most intensity when it is applied right on top of soft pencil eyeliner. Just dab it on, never rub it in. It is better to use a brush or applicator here than your fingertip. Your own eye colour will be intensified if you line the inner rim with white pencil eyeliner.

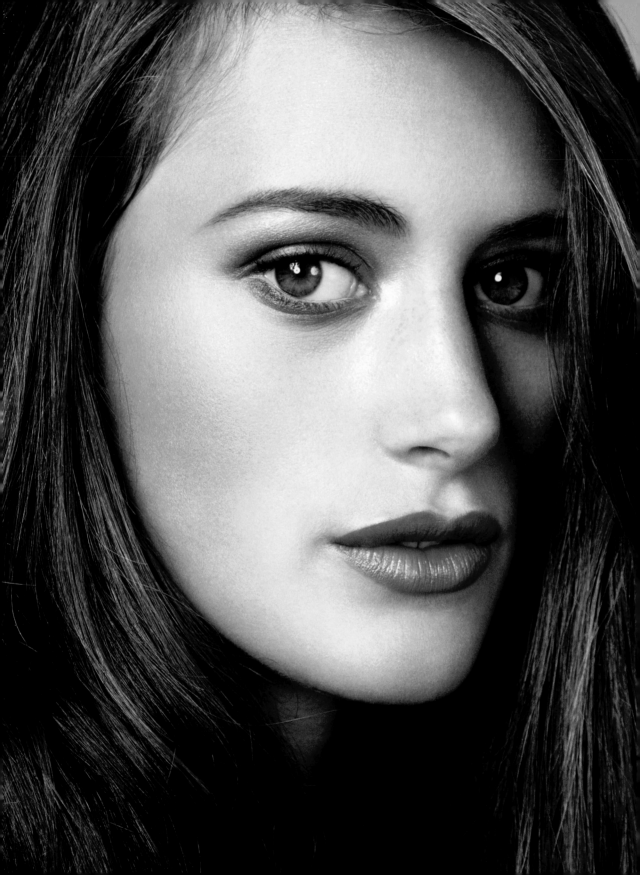

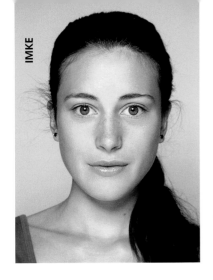

IMKE

Your eye colour always pops out when you circle your eye with eyeshadow and set the eyeshadow's highest point above the centre of the pupil.

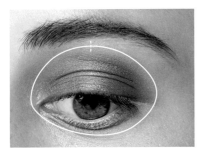

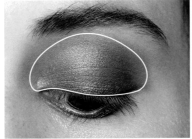

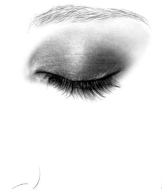

1. EYESHADOW
Completely circle the eye with copper eyeshadow. The highest point of the eyeshadow should lie above the centre of the pupil.

2. SHADING
Apply brown eyeshadow to the upper lid along the lash line. The two shades should flow seamlessly into one another.

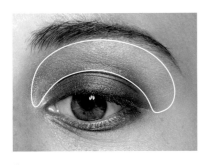

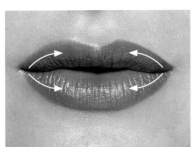

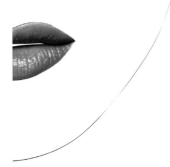

3. HIGHLIGHTS
Now apply pale eyeshadow from the lid crease upwards to the arch of the brow. Blend it in especially well at the corners of the eyes; there should be no sharp edges.

4. LIPSTICK
Apply lipstick carefully with a small, rounded brush. Always work from the corners of the mouth to the centre.

YOU WILL NEED:

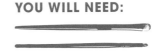

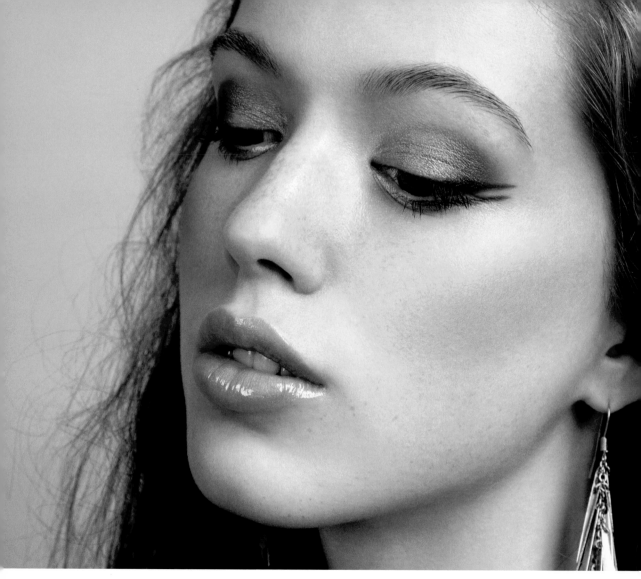

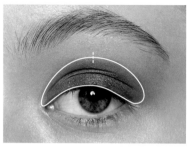

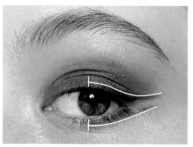

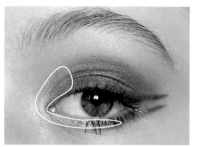

1. EYESHADOW

Apply eyeshadow over the upper lid. To give the eye a beautiful shape, the highest point of the eyeshadow should lie right above the centre of the pupil.

2. PENCIL EYELINER

Using a soft pencil eyeliner, and starting just above the pupil, draw a line along the upper and lower lash lines. Extend the lines beyond the outer corner of the eye.

3. MASCARA

The mascara, too, is applied to the upper and lower lashes just from the centre of the eye to the outer corner of the eye. The inner corner of the eye is accented with highlighter.

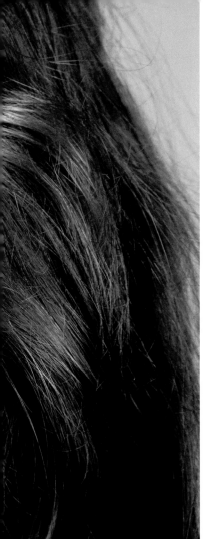

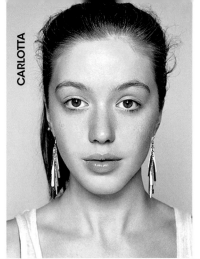

CARLOTTA

/**TIP:** Do you want plumper lips? By using lip gloss, you can make the lips seem fuller. This is easy to do. After applying lipstick, dab a matching colour of gloss on the centre of your lips. So that the lip gloss remains within the lip line, do not bring it right up to the lip line.

YOU WILL NEED:

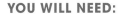

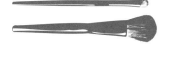

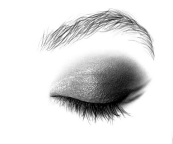

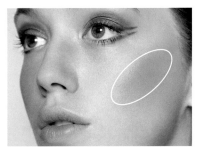

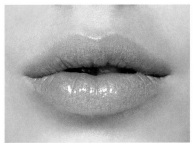

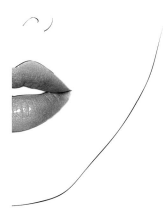

4. BLUSHER

Blusher is applied to the centre of the cheekbone and blended out to all sides. This gives soft edges.

5. GLOSS

A lip gloss with shiny particles best matches the shimmery eyeshadow.

SINA

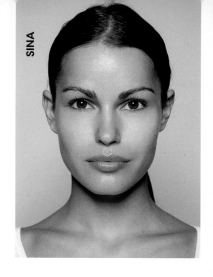

YOU WILL NEED:

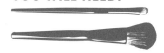

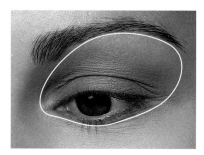

1. EYESHADOW
Circle the entire eye with eyeshadow, bringing it up to underneath the brow. Make sure the eyeshadow colour is even overall.

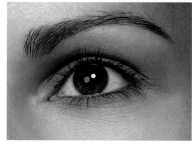

2. MASCARA
Mascara is a must if you want to emphasize your eyes. First, apply mascara to the fine hairs at the inner and outer corners of the eye, then to the upper and lower lashes.

/**TIP:** You don't really need a cupboard full of products to achieve a good look. To create this style of make-up, you can also use the eyeshadow as a blusher and a lipstick. All that's missing is the mascara – then the look is ready.

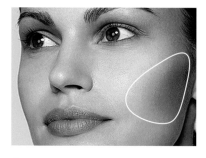

3. OUTLINE
For a fresh look, and also to accentuate the cheekbone, put a bit of eyeshadow on your blusher brush, apply it just under your cheekbone, and blend it in.

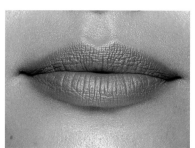

4. LIPS
Apply lip balm to your lips and then, using your fingertip, dab on a bit of eyeshadow.

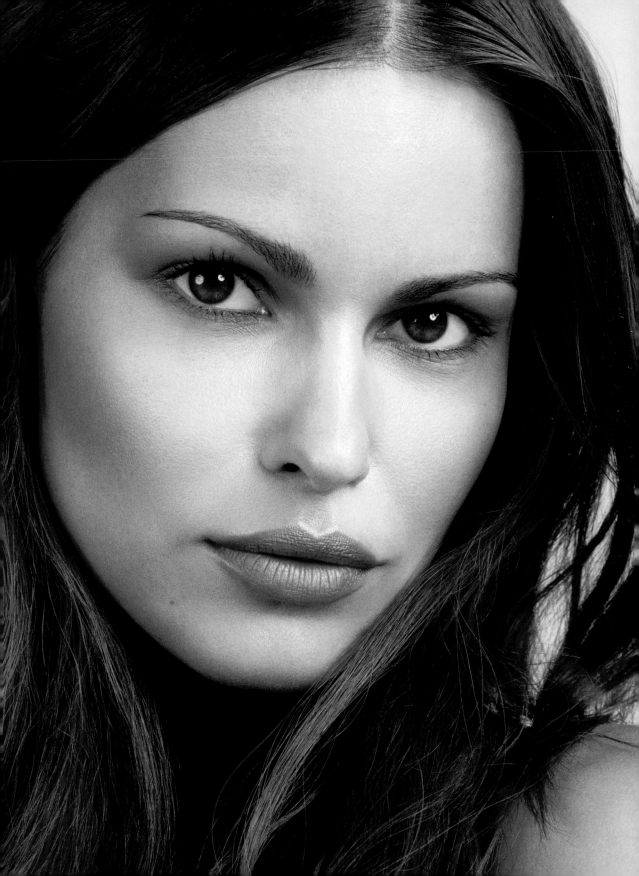

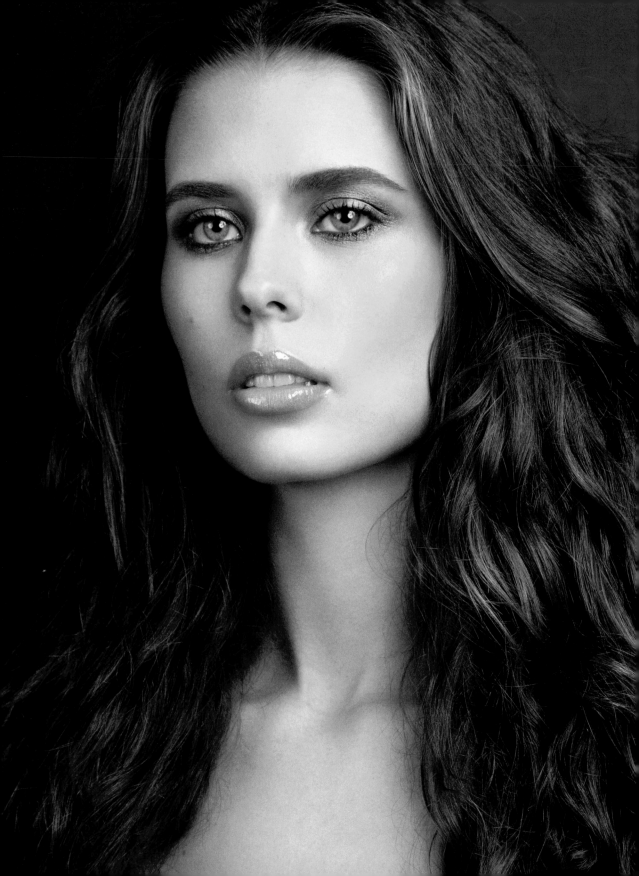

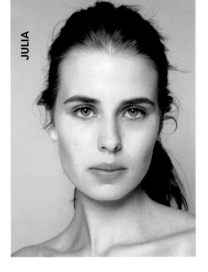

JULIA

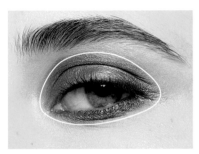

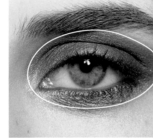

YOU WILL NEED:

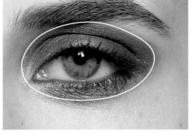

1. CIRCLE

Circle your eye with an iridescent grey tone. Make sure that the eyeshadow meets at the inner and outer corners of the eye.

2. SECOND COLOUR

Brush gold eyeshadow over the grey upwards all the way to the brow line. Apply the gold shadow to the lower lash line, working from the inner to the outer corner of the eye.

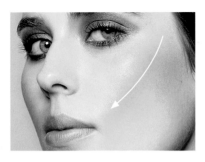

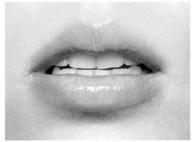

3. BLUSHER & MASCARA

Using a foundation brush, apply cream blusher to the highest point of the cheekbone and then downward to the corner of the mouth. Then coat your eye lashes with mascara.

4. LIPS

Now the only thing left to do is to apply pastel-coloured lip gloss and the make-up is done.

/**TIP:** Shimmery, glittery, or glossy? These lipstick textures reflect the light perfectly, fill out little lip creases, and thus make lips look plumper. This is also why shimmery and glittery eyeshadow makes the eyes look younger.

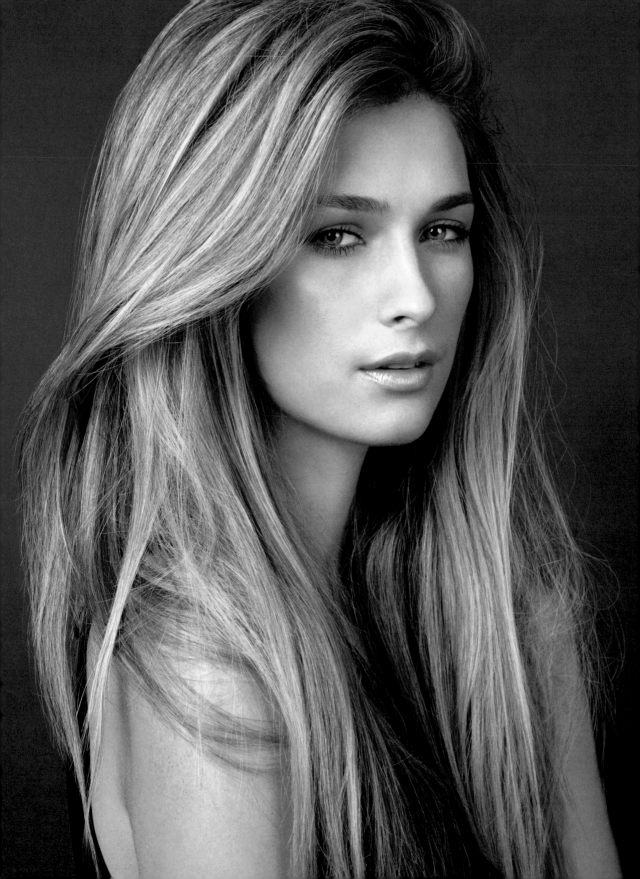

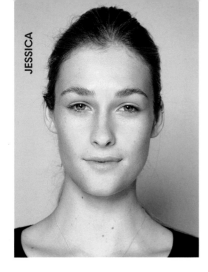

JESSICA

For this make-up style, the face is contoured and emphasis given to the eyes. Pink makes for a cool and modern look. If this seems too extreme to you, you can use another shade of blusher for this look.

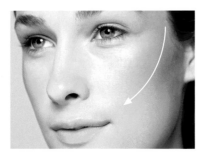

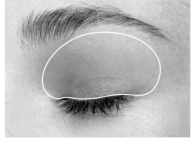

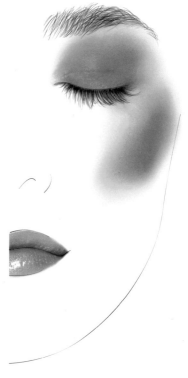

1. OUTLINE
Using a blusher brush, brush the eyeshadow downwards from the temple. With your finger, blend the edges downwards towards the corners of your mouth.

2. LID
Apply eyeshadow over the upper lid all the way up to the brow line. Start at the lash line and blend out softly.

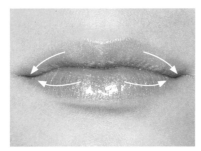

3. EYELASHES & PENCIL EYELINER
Apply pencil eyeliner to the inner rim of the eye. Then, apply layers of mascara to upper and lower lashes.

4. LIPS
Apply shiny, nude gloss to the centre of your lips. Smooth it out to all sides.

YOU WILL NEED:

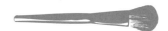

BASIC TECHNIQUES: EYES

Make-up is fantastic for correcting little imperfections. By following these simple tips, hooded eyes, small eyes, wide-set, and close-set eyes can be easily disguised with eyeshadow.

YOU WILL NEED:

YOU WILL NEED:

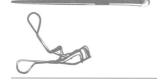

1. HOODED EYES

Apply highlighter directly underneath the brow. Using a larger, rounded brush, apply eyeshadow on the eye crease, following the curve of the lid. This ensures the entire hooded lid is covered. It is important that the eyeshadow is visible when the eye is open.

2. SMALL EYES

Apply highlighter directly underneath the brow. Now work with light-reflecting eyeshadows. Use a paler shade on the upper lid and a darker one on the eye crease. Then curl your eyelashes. This opens up the eye and makes it seem larger. Apply mascara to the upper and lower lashes.

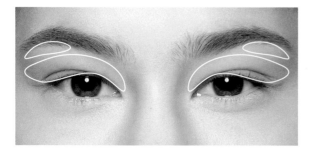

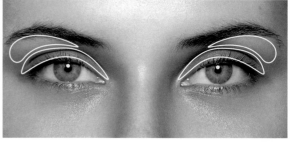

/TIP: Light colours have little effect. The darker the eyeshadow, the better the result.

/TIP: It is easy to enlarge small eyes. Carefully blend in the edges of the two shades of eyeshadow to avoid hard lines.

3. CLOSE-SET EYES

If you have close-set eyes, the inner corner of the eye should be accented with paler eyeshadow and the outer corner of the eye emphasized with darker eyeshadow. The eyeshadow should be blended around the outside of the eyes – this lengthens the eye visually.

4. WIDE-SET EYES

Apply dark eyeshadow sparingly to the inner corner of the eye in the shape of a horizontal "v". Blend out the eyeshadow on the upper lid. Using the same colour, lightly shade in the outer corner of the eye. Apply highlighter under the outer third of the eyebrow. Then, apply mascara to the upper and lower lashes.

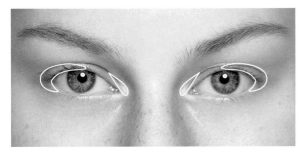

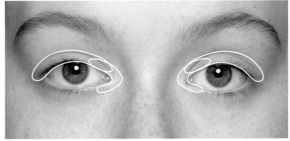

/**TIP:** The closer you get to the bridge of the nose, the softer and lighter the colour should be.

/**TIP:** By applying darker pencil eyeliner to the inner rims, the eyes seem to be pushed closer together.

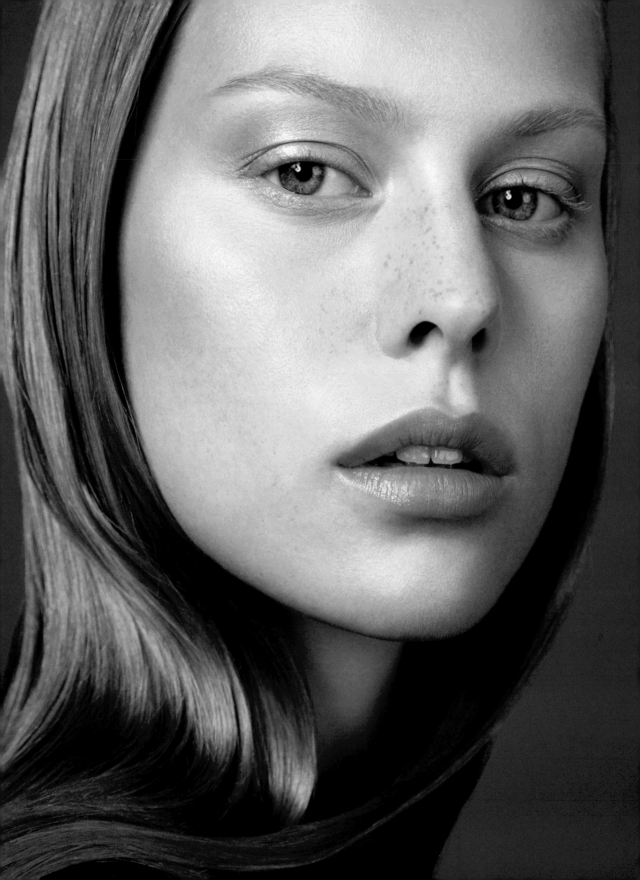

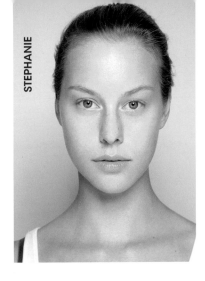

Shape, intensity, and colour – these building blocks make the look. When you are experimenting with eyeshadow, do play with various colour intensities. If the shape is good, and the intensity of colour is even, every look is great.

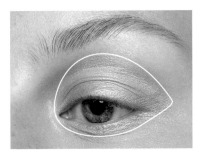

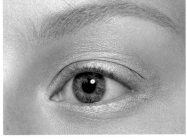

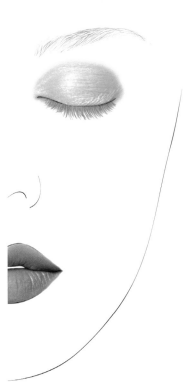

1. EYESHADOW
Completely encircle your eye with pastel green eyeshadow. A large eyeshadow brush makes an easy job of blending-in any hard edges.

2. EYEBROWS
To get a subtle look such as this, the eyebrow must be understated. Dab a thin layer of foundation on the eyebrow and blend in the edges with a small eyebrow brush.

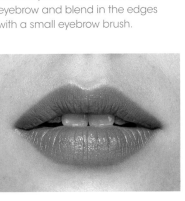

3. MASCARA & PENCIL EYELINER
Comb the eyelashes. Apply nude mascara, then dot green eyeshadow on the eyelashes. Apply coloured pencil eyeliner to the inner rim.

4. LIP BALM
Just a light, natural shimmer should be seen on the lips. All you need to do to get this effect is to dab on a bit of lip balm.

YOU WILL NEED:

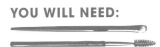

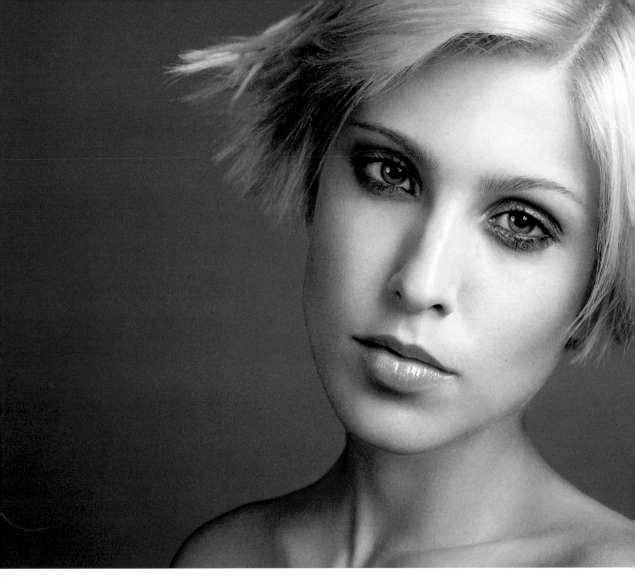

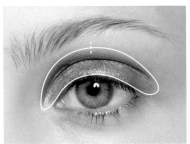

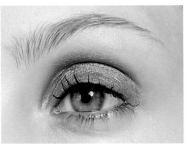

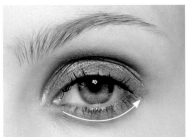

1. EYESHADOW

Using a large, rounded brush, apply enough eyeshadow so that the colour is just barely visible when the eye is open. In this look, too, the highest point of the eyeshadow is set right above the pupil.

2. MASCARA

Gently curl your eyelashes so that the eye looks larger and wide-awake. Then, using a gentle zigzag motion, liberally layer the eyelashes with black mascara from the bottom of the lash line to the tips.

3. SECOND EYESHADOW

Grey eyeshadow is a great complementary colour to this vibrant blue. Using a rounded brush, evenly apply the grey eyeshadow along the lower lash line.

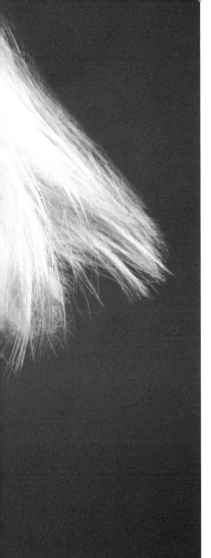

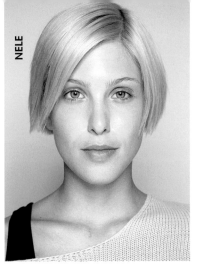

NELE

/TIP: When you use intense colours like this brilliant turquoise, a neutral colour, such as grey, is the perfect complement. Grey makes the make-up look more balanced; the bright colour doesn't dominate quite as much.

YOU WILL NEED:

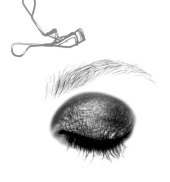

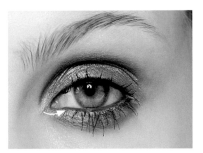

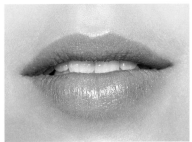

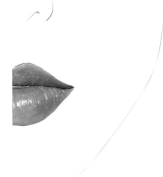

4. PENCIL EYELINER

Pick an eyeliner pencil colour that matches the grey eyeshadow. Draw a line from the inner to the outer corner of the eye. Finally, apply mascara to the lower lashes.

5. LIPS

So that nothing detracts from the luminous eyes, apply just a bit of lip balm to the lips.

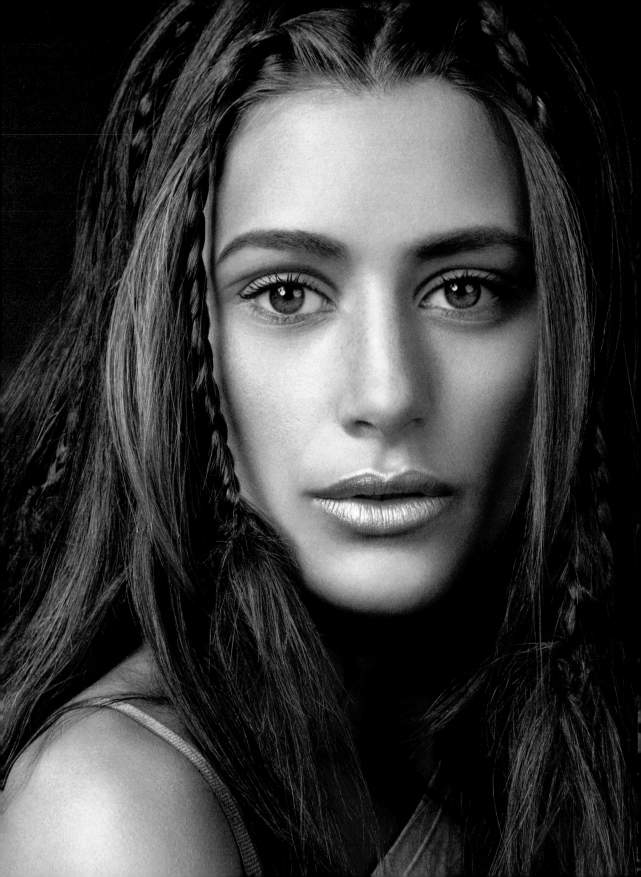

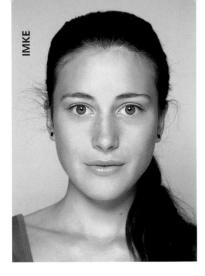

IMKE

YOU WILL NEED:

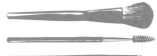

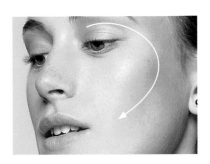

1. OUTLINE

Use bronzing powder to create contour. Apply bronzer over the upper lid from the inner to the outer corner of the eye. Blend it downwards to the cheekbone and along the chin.

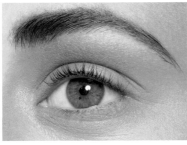

2. EYEBROWS

First, brush the eyebrows into shape. Then, using an eyebrow pencil, trace along the brows.

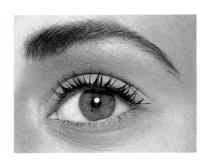

3. EYELASHES

Apply several layers of mascara to the upper lashes. Use blue mascara on the lower lashes to set a highlight.

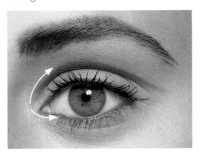

4. LID

Starting at the inner corner, apply blue pencil eyeliner to the inner rim of your eye. Then, with your eye open, draw a beautiful arch just above the eye crease.

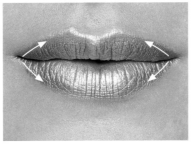

5. LIPS

Draw the lip outline with gold cream eyeshadow. Then, dab eyeshadow on the lips.

/TIP: Even if you don't have any blue mascara on hand, you can create a similar effect with nude mascara and blue eyeshadow. Simply apply a layer of mascara to the bottom lashes and carefully brush on the blue eyeshadow. If you would like to use other colours of mascara for this look, there is no reason not to!

BASIC TECHNIQUES: PENCIL EYELINER

Pencil eyeliner can be used to create many different looks. It is fabulous as a base for smokey eyes. Whatever the look, just make sure the eyeliner is soft and oily; otherwise you will not be able to duplicate this technique.

/BLACK
For more definition

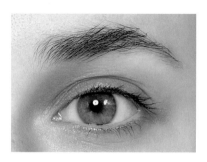 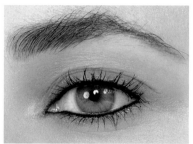

BEFORE
Applying black to the inner rim frames and shapes the eyes. Always apply eyeliner to the inner corner of the eye so that the eye appears round and almond-shaped.

AFTER
Even if the eye loses definition with age, applying black pencil eyeliner to the inner rim can make the eyes seem younger.

/WHITE
For sparkling eyes

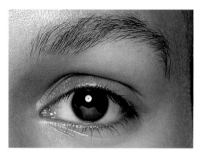 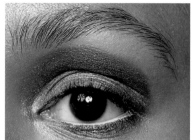

BEFORE
White pencil eyeliner makes the eye look larger and the white of the eye clearer. This is a great trick to make your eyes look alert again, especially when they are a bit red!

AFTER
Be careful here. Use pencil eyeliner sparingly since otherwise you can quickly end up with an Eighties look.

Waterproof pencil eyeliners let you create very diverse looks. They also allow you to work with great accuracy.

/BLUE

As a complementary colour

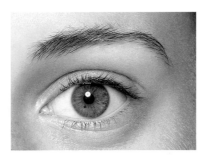

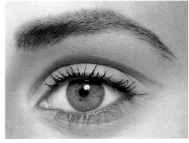

BEFORE
When coloured pencil eyeliner is used as a complementary colour, it will intensify your own eye colour and make it stand out.

AFTER
Coloured pencil eyeliner can serve as a base for tone-on-tone shading, too. If you use blue pencil eyeliner as a base for blue eyeshadow, the colour will be especially intense.

/BROWN

For gentle, smokey eyes

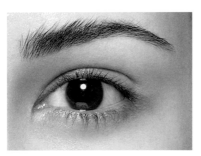

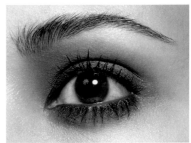

BEFORE
Brown goes well with warm eye colours and makes the eyes look soft. Cool eye colours such as blue, grey-blue, and grey-green look more intense when you use brown pencil.

AFTER
Unlike black, brown reflects light, so brown is a good base for a variety of eyeshadow colours.

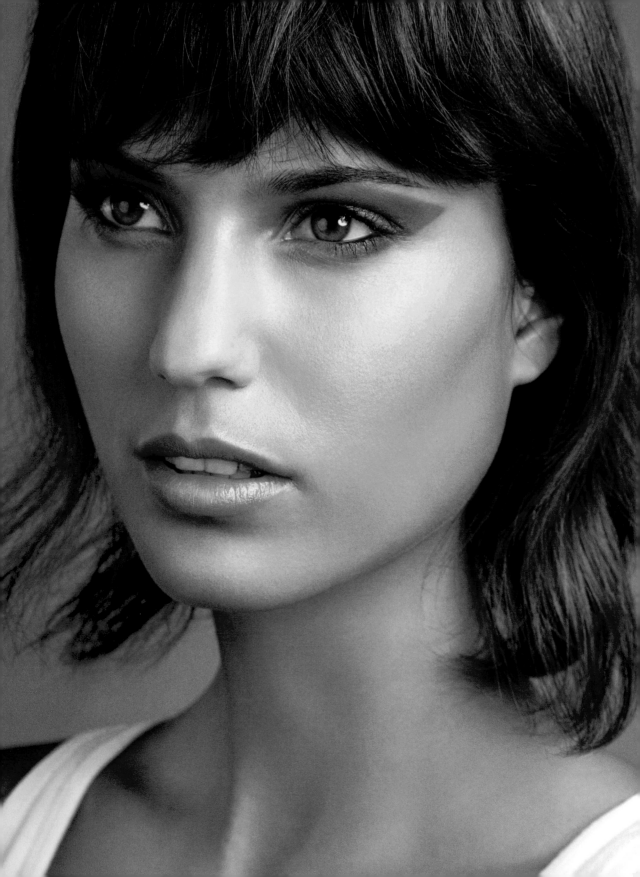

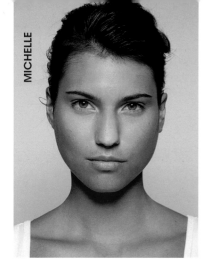

MICHELLE

This look has been kept very soft by using two shades of brown. You can choose more intense colours for an evening out.

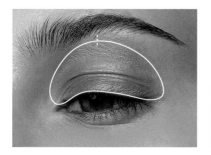

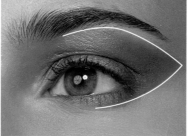

YOU WILL NEED:

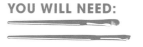

1. EYESHADOW

Using a small, rounded brush, apply eyeshadow over the upper lid, blending it up to the brow line at the highest point above the pupil.

2. SECOND EYESHADOW

Using a darker shade and an angled brush, extend the eyeshadow out beyond the eye in the shape of a triangle. Start on the outer side of the pupil and work out above and below the eye.

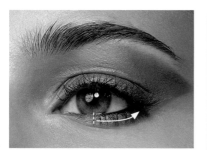

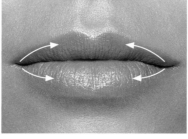

3. EYELASHES & PENCIL EYELINER

For a smouldering look, apply pencil eyeliner to the inside rim from the outer corner of the eye to the pupil. Apply mascara to the lower lashes only as far as the line extends.

4. LIPSTICK

Carefully apply lipstick using a small, rounded lipstick brush. Always work from the corners of the mouth to the centre.

/**TIP:** When you work with pencil eyeliner, don't forget to apply eyeliner to the little "v" in the inner and outer corners of the eye. This makes the eye look almond-shaped. But, if your eyes are wide-set, emphasize just the outer corners of the eyes. This will make the eyes look as though they are closer together.

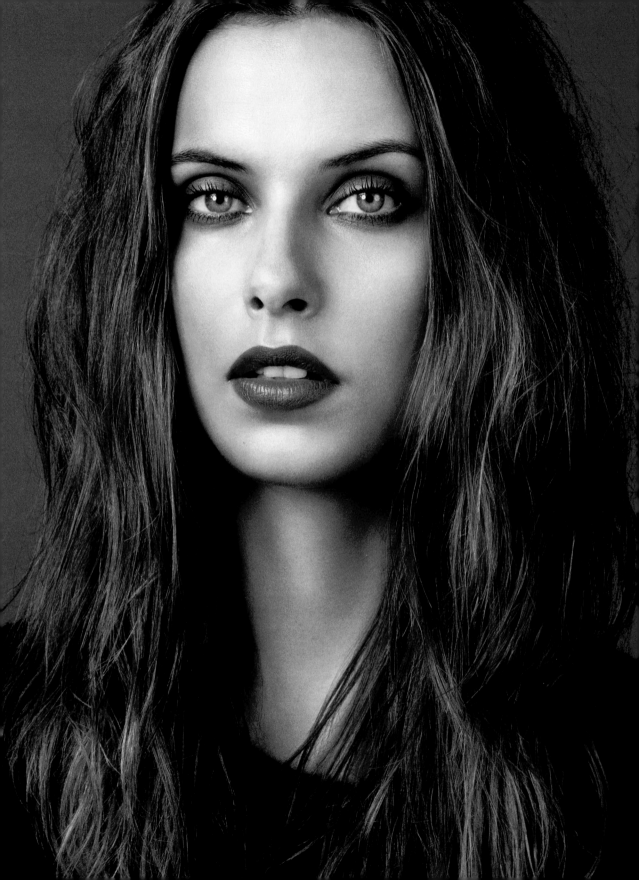

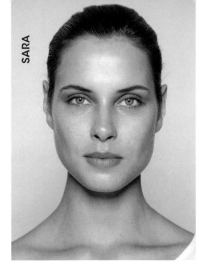

SARA

This look is sexy and seductive with its smokey eyes and dark lips.

/ **TIP:** Don't forget to spend some time on your eyebrows when your eyes are heavily emphasized. Pluck out the little fine hairs. Then, brush the eyebrows into shape with an eyebrow brush. This will direct further attention to the eyes.

YOU WILL NEED:

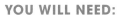
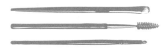

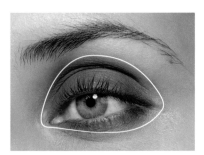

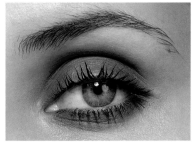

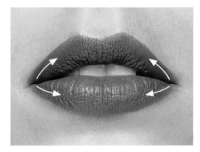

1. EYESHADOW

Using a wide, rounded eyeshadow brush, apply eyeshadow over the entire upper lid. Make sure that the most intense eyeshadow colour is applied along the lower lash line.

2. MASCARA

First, free the eyelashes of bits of stray eyeshadow with a small brush. Then, apply layers of mascara to the upper and lower lashes. The mascara should be thickest along the lash lines. Brush the eyebrows well.

3. LIPSTICK

Beautiful dark lips complement smokey eyes wonderfully. Here, first draw the outline carefully and then fill in the lips.

BASIC TECHNIQUES: EYELASHES

Start with the most difficult task – apply mascara to the fine hairs at the inner corner of the eye, then to the longer hairs at the outer corner. Then, focus on the lash lines. Finally, run the wand over the lashes and tips. This makes a big difference.

YOU WILL NEED:

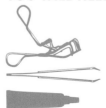

/APPLY MASCARA PERFECTLY

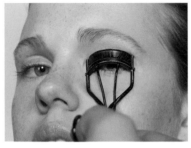

1. PLACING

Eyelash curlers that have a soft rubber cushion prevent the lashes from breaking. Place the curler on the upper lash line and squeeze.

2. CURLING

Open the eyelash curler and pull it halfway down the length of the lashes. Squeeze firmly. Repeat. This gives the eyelashes a great sweep.

3. APPLYING MASCARA

Apply mascara in a zigzag motion, working from the bottom of the lash line to the tips. Work from the outer to the inner corner of the eye, taking care to coat the fine hairs in the corner of the eye with mascara.

/FALSE EYELASHES

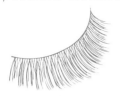

1. Classic natural-length lashes.

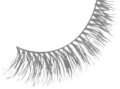

2. Thick lashes for more volume.

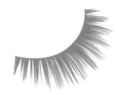

3. Natural length, fuller lashes.

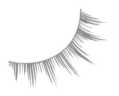

4. Extra-long lashes for a fuller look.

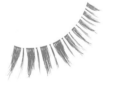

5. Thick lashes for a touch of glamour.

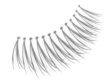

6. Indivdual lashes to add volume discreetly.

/Tip: You may wish to use tweezers to hold false eyelashes in position as you apply them. Since false eyelashes are already full, perfectly curled, and well separated, you don't need to apply any mascara to them. If they are well cared-for, false eyelashes can be reused several times without problem. Just make sure to carefully remove all the lash glue, using a pair of tweezers if needed. Store the lashes in the container they came in until they are next needed.

Use only special lash glue to apply false eyelashes. It dries quickly, is easy on the skin, adheres well, and yet can be removed easily from the false eyelashes.

/EYELASH-STYLES

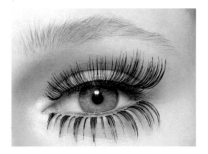

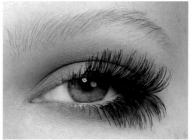

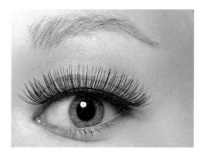

/FASHION
For a trendy look, false eyelashes also can be appled to the lower lid.

/SIXTIES
For a wonderful Sixties-look, the eyelashes are trimmed and applied to the outer corners of the eye.

/CLASSIC
These long and full eyelashes are just perfect for that seductive eyelash flutter.

/STEP-BY-STEP

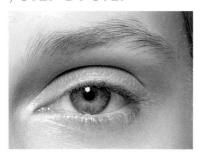

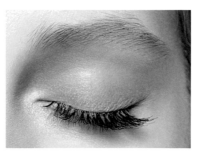

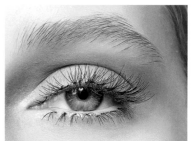

1. PREPARE
Before the eyelashes are glued on, your own eyelashes have to be curled with an eyelash curler. Don't forget the tiny fine hairs.

2. GLUE ON
Apply a small amount of glue to the base of the false lashes. Blow on the glue a bit so it becomes sticky. Now position the lashes at the centre of the lash line.

3. LET DRY
Press gently on the lashes and let them dry for a few seconds. The false lashes should extend beyond the ends of your natural lashes.

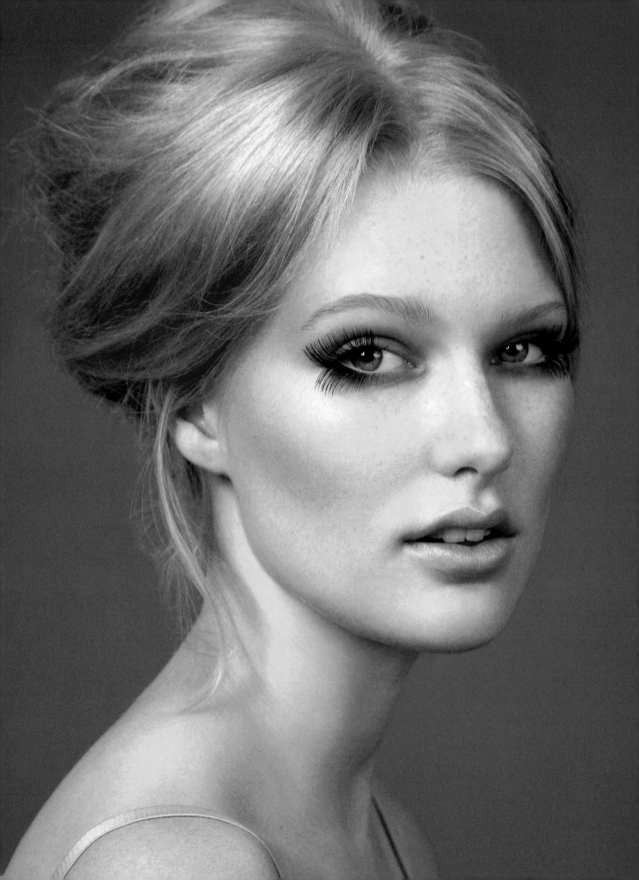

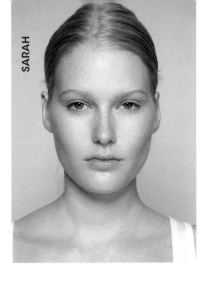

SARAH

False lashes are easy to remove with eye make-up remover. If you carefully pack the lashes away (after first freeing them of glue) you can re-use them several times without any problems.

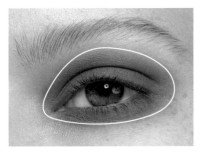

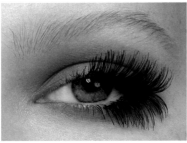
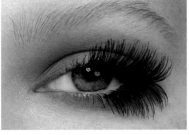

YOU WILL NEED:

1. EYESHADOW

Circle your eye with a light, matte eyeshadow. Apply the eyeshadow with a large brush and blend in the edges.

2. FALSE EYELASHES

For a Sixties-look, emphasize just the outer lashes. Trim false eyelashes to the desired width and glue them on, using tweezers to help position them.

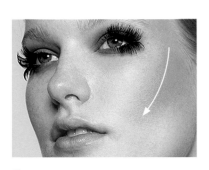

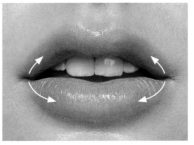

/**TIP:** You can set great accents with false eyelashes. For this particular look, it is crucial that the upper and lower lashes don't touch. Also, if the false eyelashes extend too far beyond the outer corner of the eye, the eye will look sad.

3. BLUSHER

For a perfect retro-look, apply a bit of apricot-coloured blusher. Start at the temple and blend in downwards and upwards towards the highest point of your cheeks.

4. LIPSTICK

The lips are covered with a soft and shimmery beige lipstick. Apply the lipstick from the corners of the mouth towards the centre.

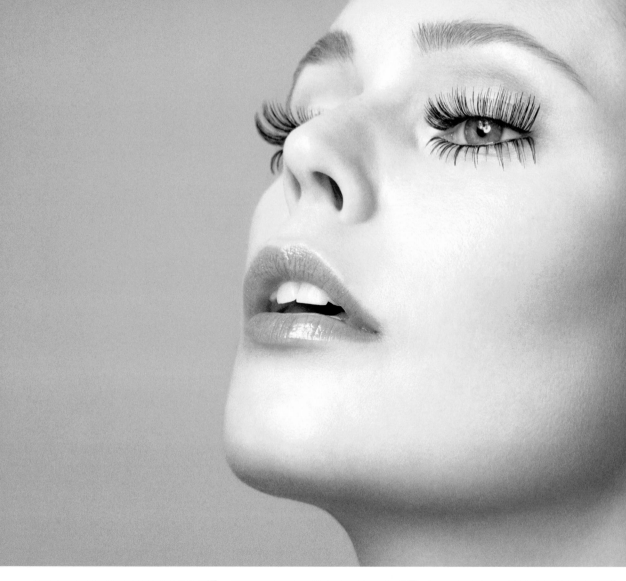

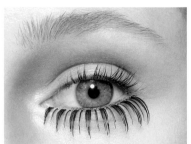

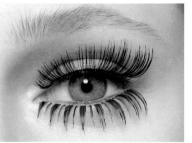

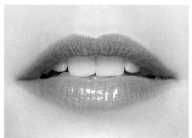

1. LOWER LID LASHES

For a dramatic look, you can also use fake eyelashes on the lower lid. Apply a thin layer of glue to the back of the lashes, let it dry a bit, and affix the lashes close to the lash line.

2. UPPER LID LASHES

Curl your own eyelashes well with an eyelash curler. Let the glue dry for a few seconds and place the lashes close to the lash line. You won't need mascara for this look.

3. LIPS

Gloss makes the lips look plumper. Here, a saturated peach tone, which goes well with fair skin, is used.

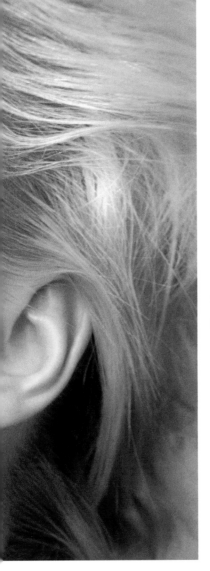

JOANA

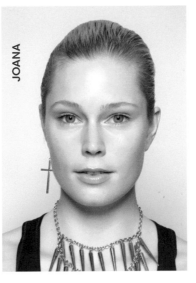

YOU WILL NEED:

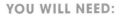
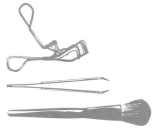

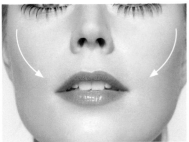

4. BLUSHER

Using a rounded brush, apply a soft blusher to the cheekbones. Blend it gently upwards to the temples and downwards towards the corners of the mouth.

/**TIP**: A delicate shade, such as peach, looks natural on a light complexion. For glamourous evening make-up, you can just as easily use intense colours. While a Snow White type can reach for a saturated red lipstick, redheads best suit orange shades. Every shade of red flatters those with darker skin tones and brown hair.

BASIC TECHNIQUES:
LIQUID EYELINER

YOU WILL NEED:

To draw a perfect eyeline, rest your finger on your cheekbone, and prop up your elbow. This helps your hand hold the brush steady and draw an even line. The eyes are easy to lengthen visually. Start the line at the inner corner of the eye and extend it beyond the outer corner. Working with liquid or gel eyeliner is tricky but, with practice, and using these tips, you will achieve the effect you want.

/TIP: Pencil eyeliner is a bit subtler and softer than liquid eyeliner. Although liquid eyeliner is harder-looking, it emphasizes the eyes more than pencil eyeliner. You will definitely need a bit of practice to get it right.

/CLASSIC

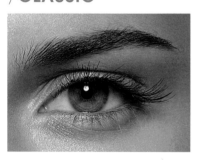 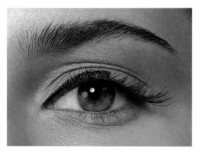 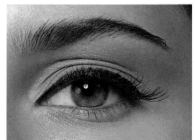

1. BASE
So that the eyeliner lasts as long as possible, dust the eye with powder. Don't use any foundation, otherwise the eyeliner will smudge immediately.

2. INNER CORNER
It is important to start the first stroke at the inner corner of the eye, otherwise the eye will look shorter.

3. OUTER CORNER
Draw a second line from the outer corner of the eye to the centre. Make sure to join the lines seamlessly where they meet.

/CAT-LIKE EYE

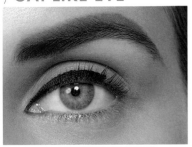

1. START
Draw the line in several strokes. Draw the first stroke along the lash line from the inner corner of the eye, ending it just to the outer side of the pupil.

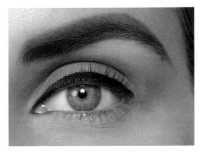

2. END
To finish the eyeline, draw a second line along the lash line from the outer corner to the centre of the pupil.

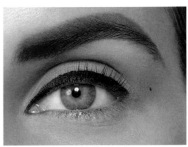

3. MARK
Decide where the "tail" should end and make a dot. End the tail above the corner of the eye, otherwise the eye will be pulled down visually.

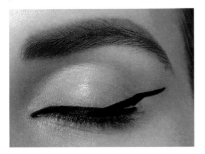

4. JOIN
Gently tighten the skin at the corner of your eye and draw a straight line from the dot to the outer side of the pupil.

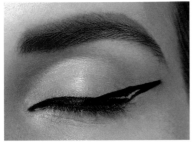

5. FILL IN
Next, connect the end of the tail with the outer corner of your eye and fill in the line. It is entirely up to you how long the winged tail should be.

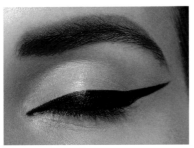

6. DRY
Do one eye first and keep it closed for a few seconds so that the eyeliner has a chance to dry.

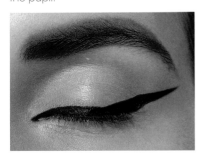

7. CORRECT
Eyeliner has to be applied perfectly. Since lopsided eyeliner ruins the symmetry of the face, carefully fill in and smooth out any rough edges.

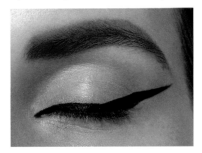

8. CONCEALER
Using a concealer brush, apply a small amount of concealer along the edges and gently brush downwards to sharpen the edges.

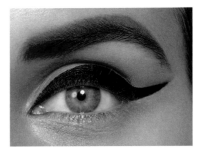

9. WOW
Eyeliner suits all those who want to emphasize their eyes. The deeper the eyeliner colour, the more intense the result.

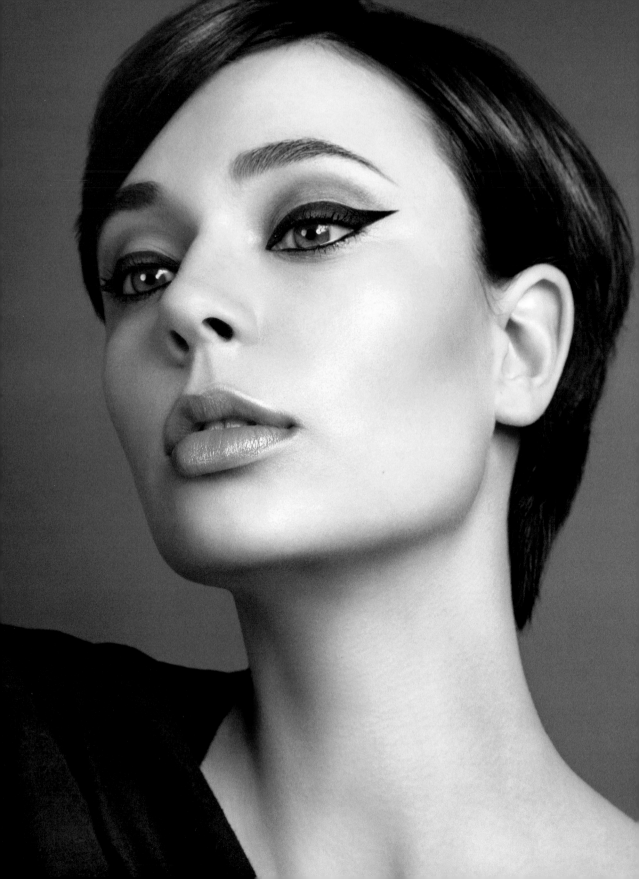

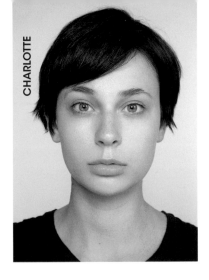

CHARLOTTE

Don't use concealer or foundation underneath eyeliner, otherwise it will smudge. You can definitely use powder and eyeshadow though.

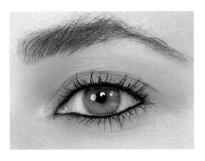

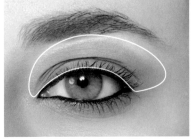

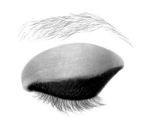

1. CIRCLE

Circle the entire inner rim with pencil eyeliner. Slightly lift up the upper lid as you are working. Then apply mascara thickly to the lashes.

2. EYESHADOW

Cover the entire upper lid with soft beige eyeshadow. Blend in the edges and check that the highest point lies above the pupil.

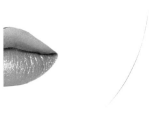

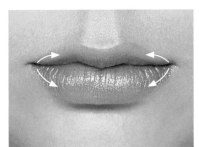

3. EYELINER

Using liquid eyeliner, draw a line in two strokes from the corners of the eye to the centre. Then, connect the end of the winged tail to the line.

4. LIPSTICK

Apply a shimmery lipstick using a brush. Always work from the corners of the lips to the centre, then carefully fill in the lips.

YOU WILL NEED:

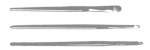

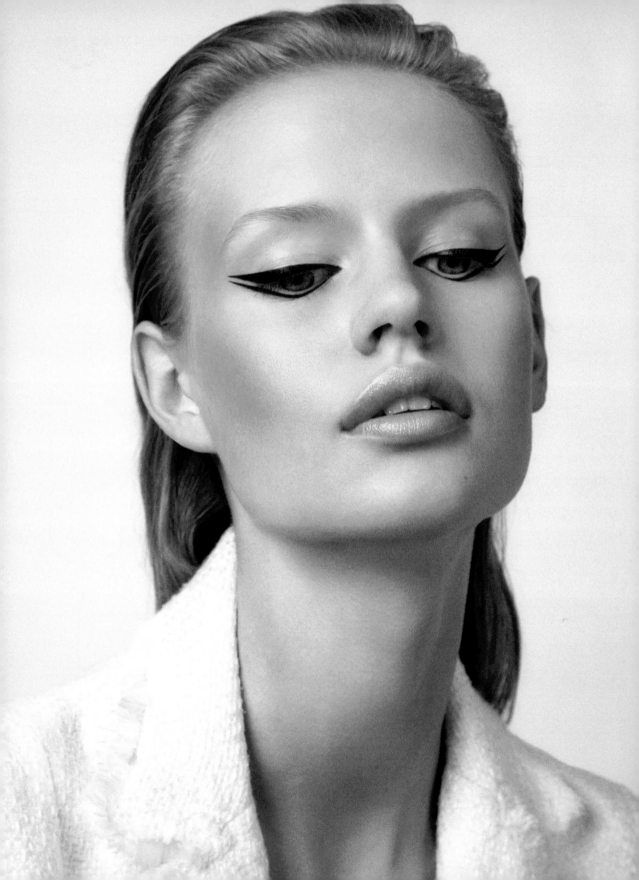

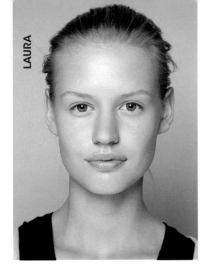

LAURA

Don't be afraid of eyeliner – with a bit of practice, using it is child's play. Just remember to start drawing the line at the inner corner of the eye, otherwise the eye will look shorter.

YOU WILL NEED:

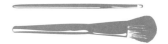

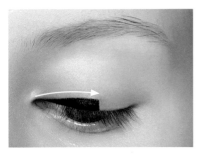

1. START DRAWING

To achieve this seductive look start by drawing a line from the inner corner of the eye to the pupil.

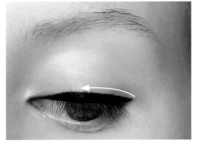

2. COMPLETE THE LINE

Next, start drawing a line just beyond the outer corner of the eye and let it meet up with the first line.

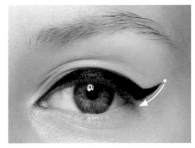

3. MAKE THE TAIL

Set a mark for the end of the winged tail above the outer corner of the eye and connect it with the eyeliner.

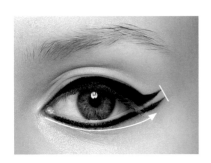

4. EYELINER

Paint a line from the lower inner corner of the eye and draw it along the lash line. Extend it out to the end of the tail. This serves to visually lengthen the eye.

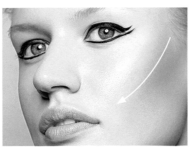

5. BLUSHER

Apply peach-coloured blusher to the cheekbone. Gently blend it upwards to the temple and downwards to the corner of the mouth.

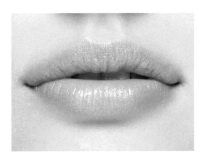

6. GLOSS

It is obvious that the eyes are the focal point of this look. All the lips need is a thin coat of gloss.

32 \ SNOW WHITE

When you use white eyeliner, your own eye colour is intensified, and your eyes look bigger.

YOU WILL NEED:

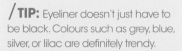

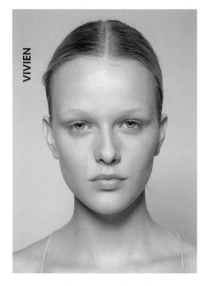

VIVIEN

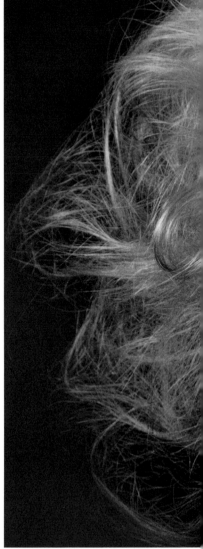

/TIP: Eyeliner doesn't just have to be black. Colours such as grey, blue, silver, or lilac are definitely trendy.

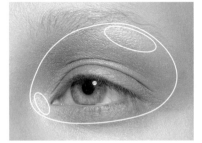

1. EYESHADOW

Circle the entire eye with eyeshadow, brushing it right up to the brow. Blend in the edges. Then, apply highlighter to the inner corner of the eye and under the brow line.

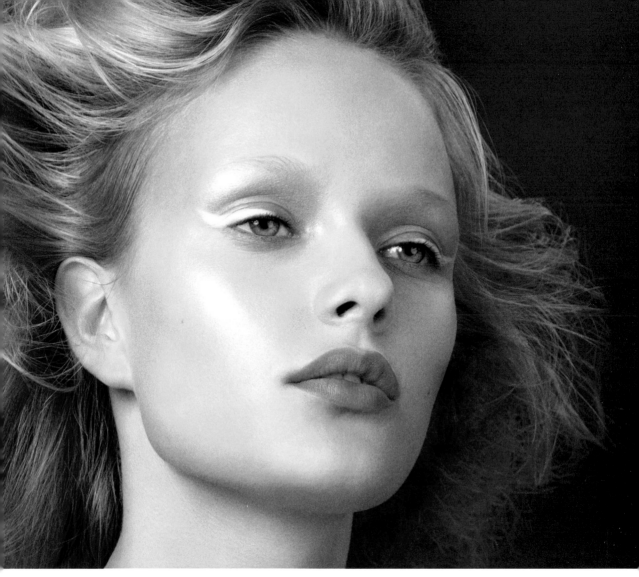

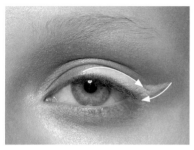

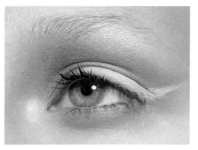

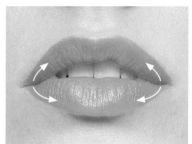

2. PENCIL EYELINER

Draw a line with a little elongated flip at the end using white pencil eyeliner. Start the line above the pupil and end it beyond the outer corner of the eye.

3. MASCARA

For a delicate, elfin look, apply a light coat of mascara to both the upper and lower lashes.

4. LIPSTICK

A delicate pink is perfect for this dreamy look. Simply apply shimmery lipstick using a lip brush and blot off the colour.

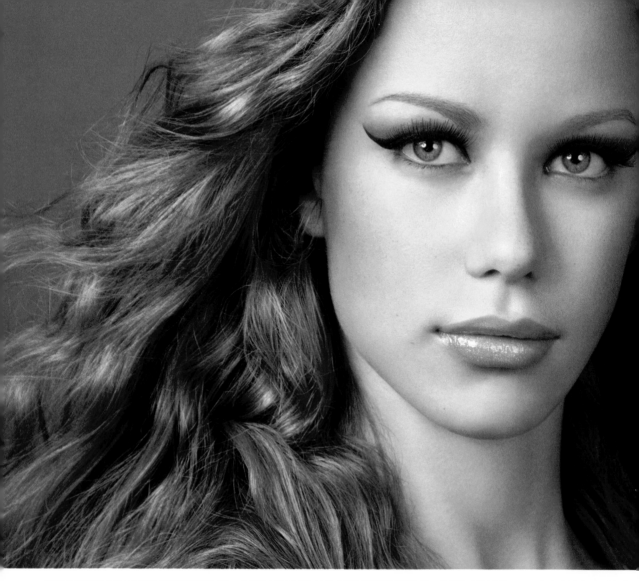

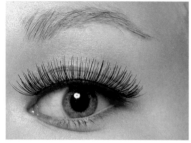

1. EYELASHES

For this highly dramatic look, you definitely need gigantic eyelashes. Follow the tips on page 82 and attach a set of fake eyelashes.

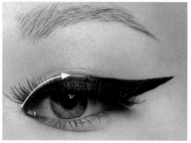

2. EYELINER

Begin the line as close to the upper lash line as possible. Draw the line from the inner to the outer corner of the eye. Then, extend the line upwards 45 degrees. Repeat several times to thicken the line.

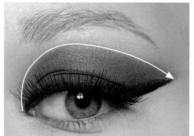

3. EYESHADOW

Apply brown eyeshadow to the upper lid, working from the inner corner of the eye to the end of the eyeliner. Continue the eyeshadow above the eye crease and upwards towards the brow.

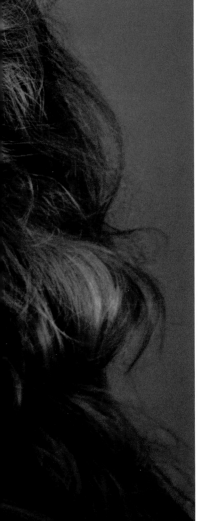

YOU WILL NEED:

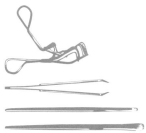

SARA

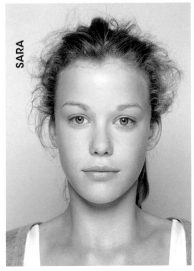

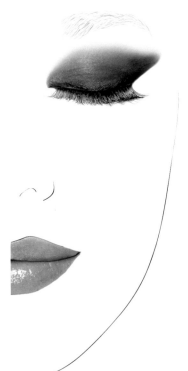

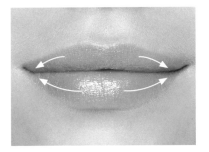

/ **TIP:** Start thickening your eyeliner gradually. This lets you slowly intensify the look. For a gentler look, apply less eyeliner or even choose a different shade. Depending on your eye shape, you can use eyeliner and shadow to create ideal almond-shaped eyes. You can also adjust for close-set or wide-set eyes. The rule of thumb is that applying a light shade to the inner corner of the eyes makes the eyes look larger. Applying a dark shade makes them look smaller.

4. **GLOSS**

Apply a thin coat of nude gloss to the centre of the top and bottom lips. Smooth it out evenly to all sides. To make the lips look larger, apply more gloss where the lips meet.

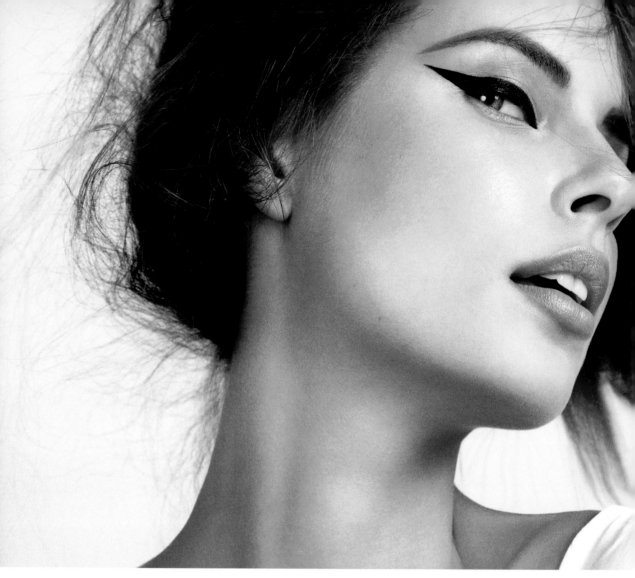

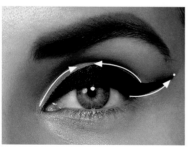

1. EYELINER

Draw the line from the inner corner of the eye to the pupil, then from the outer corner of the eye to the pupil. Now make a dot for the end of the winged tip and fill in with eyeliner.

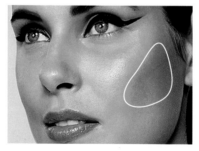

2. POWDER

Apply cream blusher before using powder. Then use translucent powder to get rid of any shiny spots on the nose, forehead, and chin.

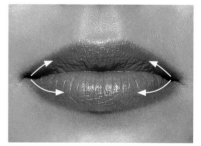

3. LIPSTICK

Using your finger, apply glossy lipstick. If you like, you can also use a lip brush.

Play with two colours of lipstick to create a jaw-dropping look.

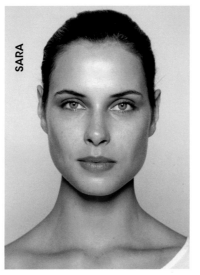

SARA

YOU WILL NEED:

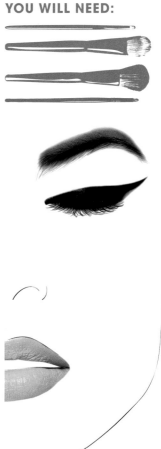

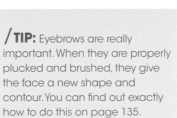

/**TIP:** Eyebrows are really important. When they are properly plucked and brushed, they give the face a new shape and contour. You can find out exactly how to do this on page 135.

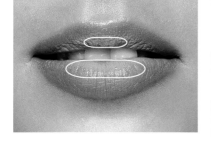

4. HIGHLIGHTS
Using a second, lighter shade of lipstick creates a great effect. Dab it on, but only apply it to the centre of your lips.

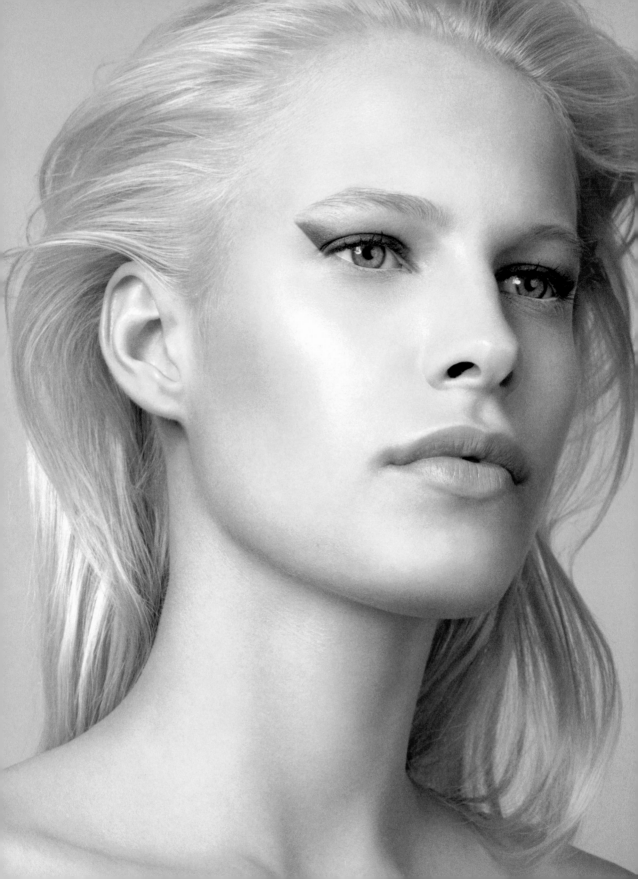

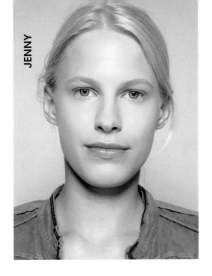

JENNY

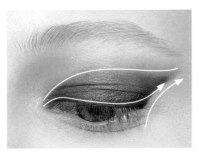

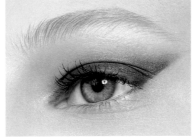
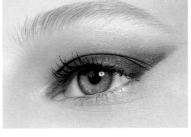

YOU WILL NEED:

1. EYE SHADOW

Using blue eyeliner, draw a line from the inner corner of the eye, extending to make a winged tip. Use an eyeshadow that matches your eyeliner and apply in the shape of a square.

2. MASCARA

Curl the eyelashes well with an eyelash curler. For even more expressive eyes, apply mascara only to the upper lashes.

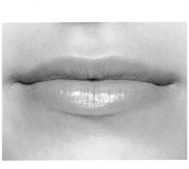
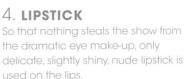

3. EYELINER

Apply skin-coloured eyeliner to the inner rim. This opens up the eye and emphasizes your eye colour.

4. LIPSTICK

So that nothing steals the show from the dramatic eye make-up, only delicate, slightly shiny, nude lipstick is used on the lips.

/**TIP:** This look is a great example of one of the countless ways you can work with eyeshadow. Eyeshadow doesn't always have to be rounded and soft. You can also use graphic shapes, as demonstrated here. Play with colour intensity to change your look bit by bit. Combine hard lines with soft shadows. Your own creativity should know no bounds – just trust yourself.

BASIC TECHNIQUES: LIPS

Only a well-sharpened lip liner creates a crisp outline. This means it is best to sharpen often!

YOU WILL NEED:

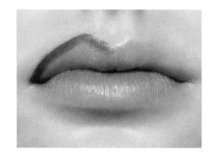

1. LEFT BOW

A perfect bow is made by working from the corner of the upper lip to the centre, which creates the desired shape.

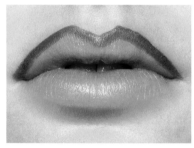

2. RIGHT BOW

The right side of the bow is created in the same way as the left. Sharpen your lip liner as you work to create a clearly defined, even outline.

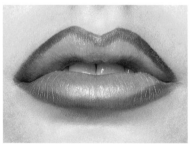

3. LOWER LIP

The outline of the lower lip is also drawn in two steps. Work from the corner of the lower lip to the centre on each side. You can correct any unevenness with lip liner at this stage.

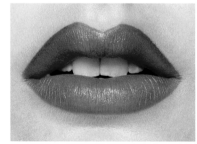

4. FILL IN

Apply the lipstick with a brush, being careful not to paint over the lip outline. Then, so the colour lasts longer, powder your lips and reapply lipstick. To finish, define the outline with concealer.

From high-sheen to extreme matte, here are six examples that show how you can accentuate your mouth and create beguiling lips.

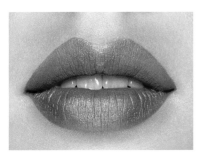

LIPSTICK

If you are using bolder colours, it is best to use a lip brush. First outline the lips from the corners of the mouth to the centre, then fill in the lips.

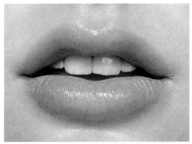

BARELY THERE

For a natural look, soft beige is ideal. Don't use a brush, just apply the lipstick directly to your lips. Always work from the corners of the mouth to the centre.

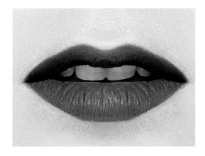

LIP LINER

Here, only lip liner is used and the lips then are blotted, powdered, and repainted with lip liner. This gives an especially long-lasting, matte result.

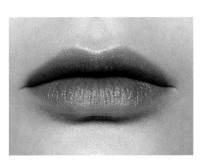

DABS OF COLOUR

An understated look is achieved by only partially applying lipstick. First, apply a bit of lip balm to your lips, close your lips, and then dab on the lipstick using your fingertip.

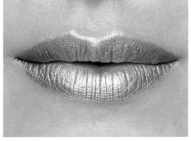

EYE SHADOW

Trace the lip contours with golden cream eyeshadow. Then dab a bit of golden eyeshadow on your lips.

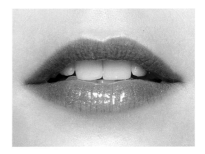

GLOSS

Lip gloss makes the lips look plumper. It is applied just like lipstick – work from the corners of the mouth to the centre.

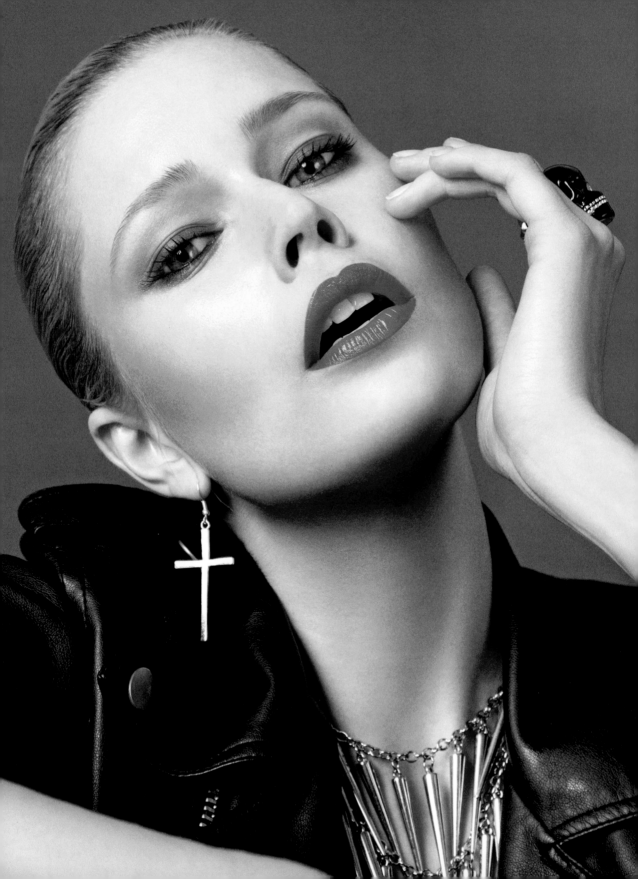

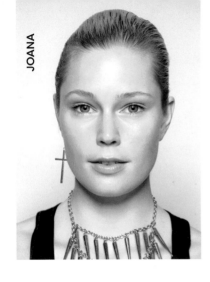
JOANA

YOU WILL NEED:

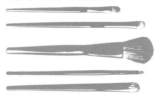

There's a perfect shade of red for every woman.
How can you find yours? Just experiment!

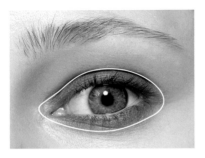

1. BASE COLOUR

Circle the eyes evenly with an intense pink shade. You will get the best results by using a smaller, rounded eyeshadow brush.

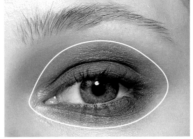

2. SECOND EYE SHADOW

Apply a light brown tone of eyeshadow with a large brush. The brown eyeshadow should fade gently into the intense pink tone.

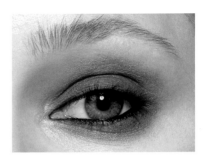

3. EYELINER

To give the eye make-up more depth, apply black pencil eyeliner over the entire inner rim.

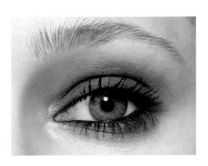

4. MASCARA

Of course, perfectly mascaraed eyes belong to this kind of look. First, apply several layers of mascara along the lash lines, then do the tips.

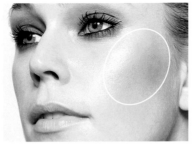

5. BLUSHER

Just a hint of colour is applied to the cheeks. Apply blusher over the entire cheekbone and gently soften upwards and downwards.

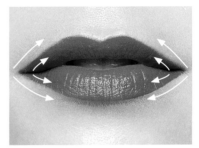

6. CLASSIC RED

Here, total accuracy is called for so use a small, angled brush to apply the red lipstick. Then, sharpen the outline with concealer.

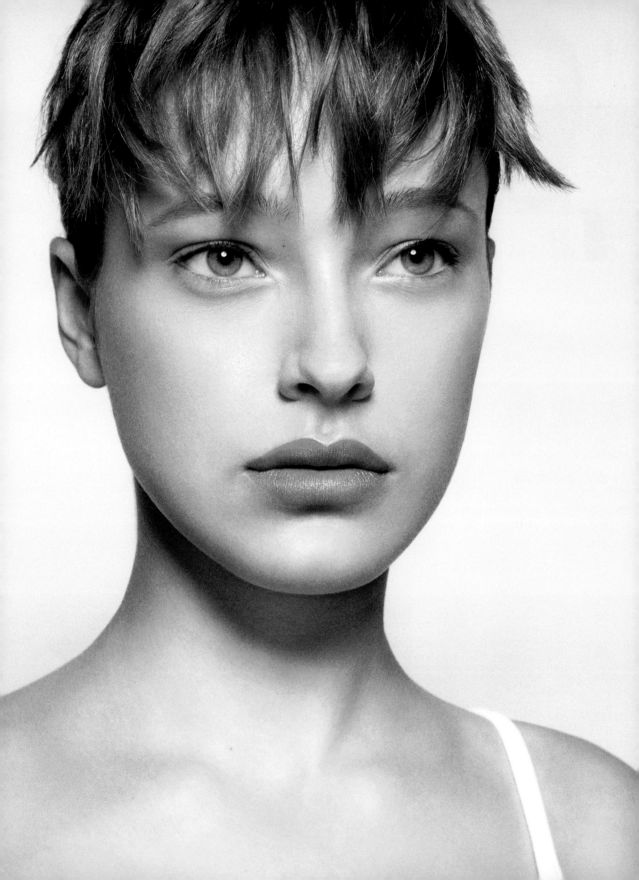

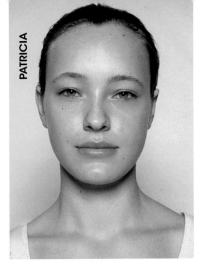

PATRICIA

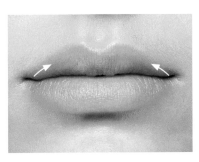

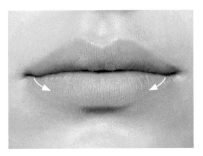

YOU WILL NEED:

1. CUPID'S BOW

Using a well-sharpened lip liner, draw the outline in two strokes from the corners to the centre of the upper lip.

2. LOWER LIP

Trace the curve of your lower lip. Your lip liner colour should match your lipstick. It is better to choose a slightly lighter shade than one that is too dark.

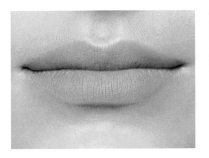

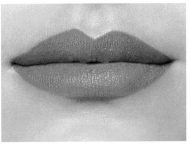

/**TIP:** Your day make-up quickly becomes suitable for an evening out with this lip look. The focus is on the lips, as the colour is intense. To make the sharpest outline, correct any unnevenness with concealer, which also serves to contour the lips.

3. FILL IN

Tighten your lips and fill them in completely with the lip liner. This creates a base for the lipstick.

4. LIPSTICK

Using a lip brush, apply the lipstick starting from the corners and working towards the centre. Take care not to paint over the outline.

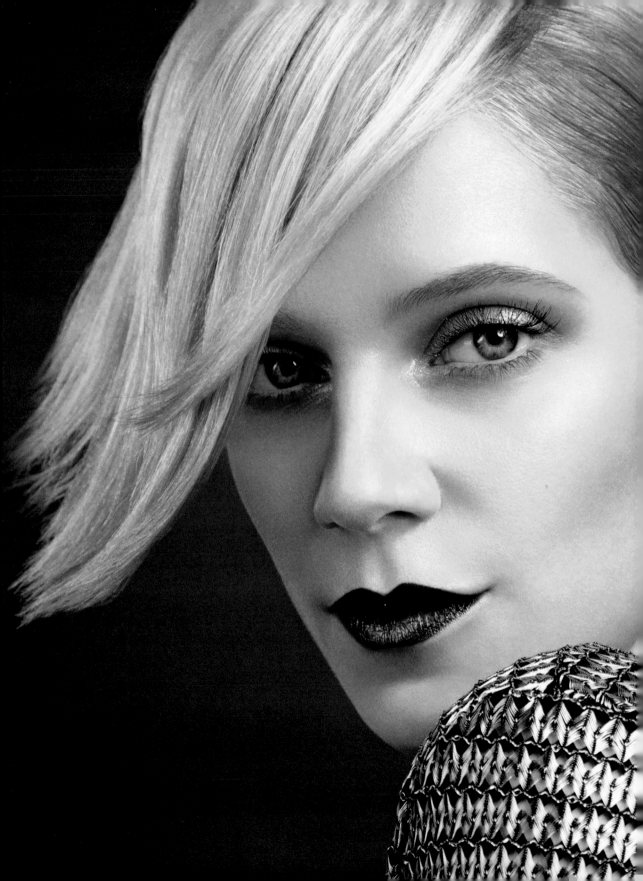

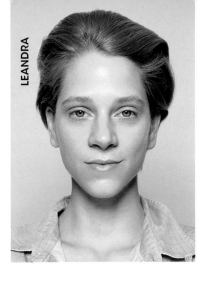

This look, with its shimmery eyeshadow and dark lips, makes you appear seductive and alluring.

/**TIP:** You can thicken your own eyelashes beautifully by applying individual false eyelashes. For the most natural look, apply the shortest lashes at the inner corner of the eye and gradually increase the lash length as you progress to the outer corner. Your eyes look wide open and your gaze electrifies. This is also an especially good and striking technique to use if you have hooded eyes.

YOU WILL NEED:

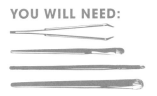

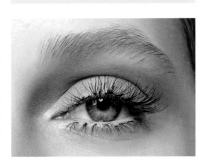

1. ADD VOLUME

For perfect, thick eyelashes, you can use individual false eyelashes. They are glued on as closely as possible to the lash line until you have the effect you want. See page 82 for more tips.

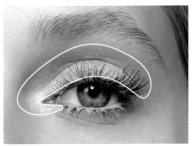

2. EYE SHADOW

Use a silver eyeshadow with shimmery particles. Start at the inner corner of the eye and apply the colour over the entire upper lid.

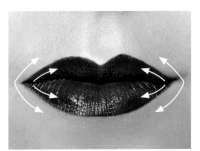

3. LIPSTICK

Using a lip brush, carefully apply the colour. Are the lips perfect? If so, apply concealer in the shape of a "v" to the corners of the mouth. This sharpens the outline.

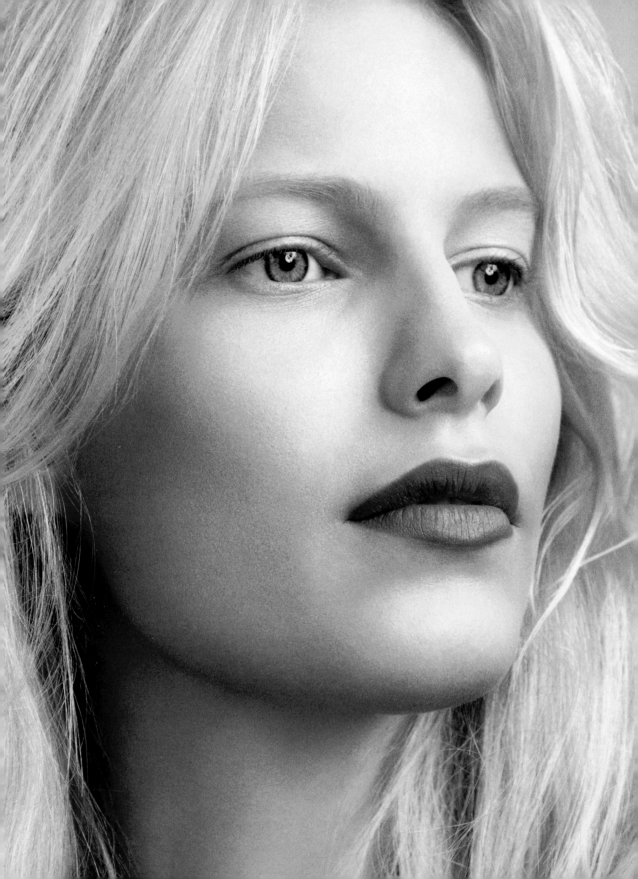

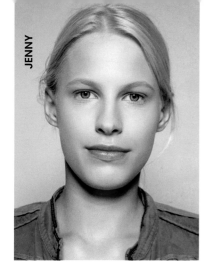

JENNY

This look is very much on trend. Nude brows are easiest to create if you have light eyebrows.

/TIP: If you don't fancy accentuating your eyebrows, you can keep them understated and instead draw attention to your lips. Downplay the eyes by using nude eyeshadow and not using any mascara.

YOU WILL NEED:

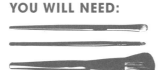

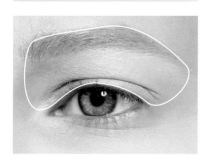

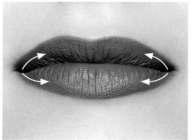

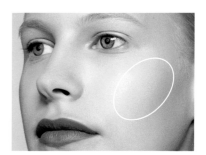

1. BROW

Understate the eyebrow by applying light eyeshadow over the entire mobile lid and above the eye crease to the top of the eyebrow. Blend in the edges especially carefully.

2. LIPSTICK

A strong brown colour on the lips suits a cool look like this one. When you are using strong colours, a well-defined outline is very important. Use a brush to apply the lipstick.

3. BLUSHER

To emphasize a fair, smooth complexion, the eyeshadow is also used as blusher. Apply eyeshadow above the temple and blend it downwards to the cheekbone.

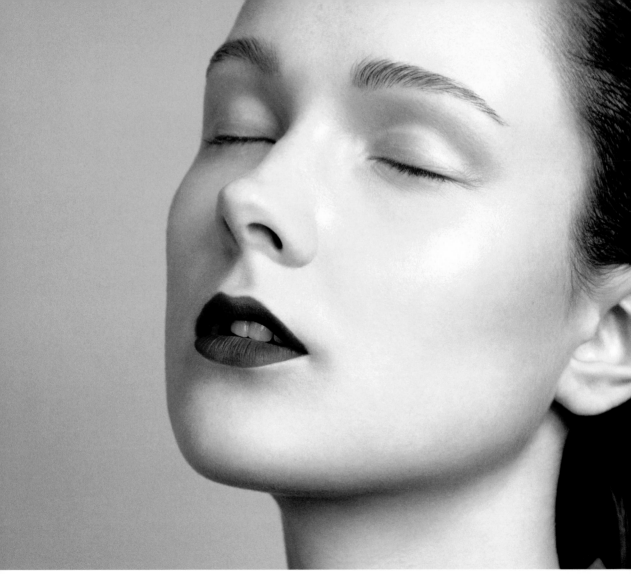

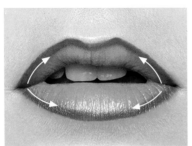

1. OUTLINE

Using a well-sharpened lip liner, draw along the contour of your lips. Always work from the corners of the mouth to the centre.

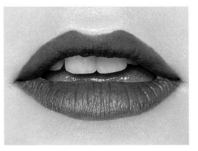

2. APPLY

Now fill in the lips with the lip liner. Work very carefully here for an even result.

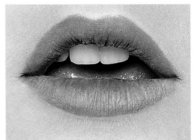

3. POWDER

To the make the colour last longer, powder your lips. Use translucent powder for this step.

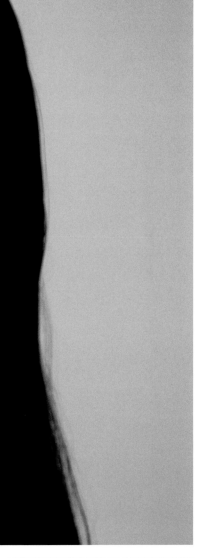

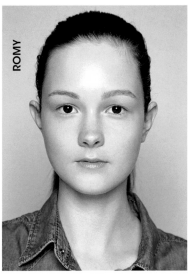

ROMY

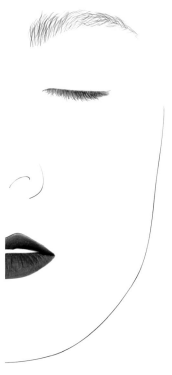

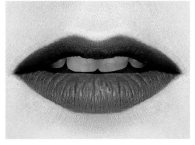

/**TIP:** We have only used lip liner here, not lipstick. For this look, it is crucial that the lip outline is perfect. After all, all eyes will be drawn to the lips. As you are applying the lip liner, keep checking to make sure that the lips look symmetrical and improve the outline as needed.

4. **APPLY**

Now apply the lip liner in the same way as in step two. This will give you the perfect matte lip look.

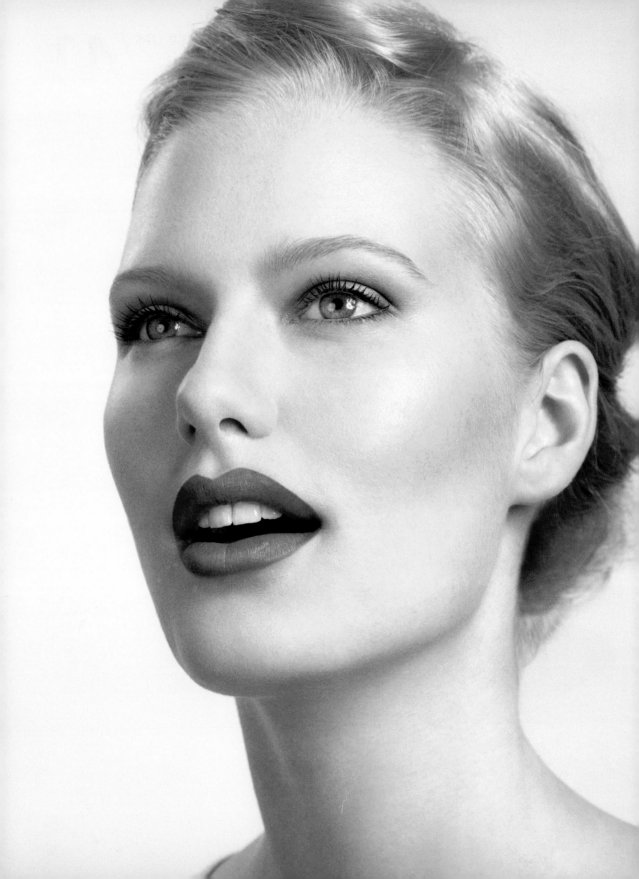

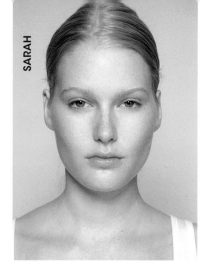

SARAH

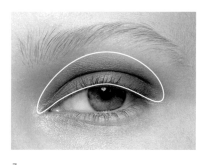

1. EYESHADOW

Apply eyeshadow over the upper lid with a rounded brush. Blend in the eyeshadow above the eye crease so the colour fades in gently up to the bottom of the brow line.

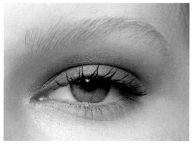

2. MASCARA

For a sensational lash look, apply several layers of mascara to the upper lashes.

YOU WILL NEED:

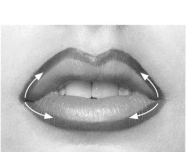

3. LIP OUTLINE

To draw the outline more easily, rest your hand on your chin. To draw an even outline, make sure you hold the pencil straight.

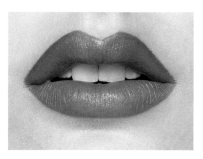

4. LIPSTICK

Carefully fill in the outline with lipstick, using a lip brush, and follow the outline precisely. Blot the lipstick, dust the lips with powder, and reapply the lipstick.

/TIP: With a bit of practice, it is easy to draw the perfect lip outline. You don't have to follow your natural lip line exactly. You can improve small imperfections with a lip brush. Since one's own lips rarely are perfect, use lip liner and lipstick to create your own ideal lip line. A perfectly shaped mouth has top and bottoms lips that are almost the same size.

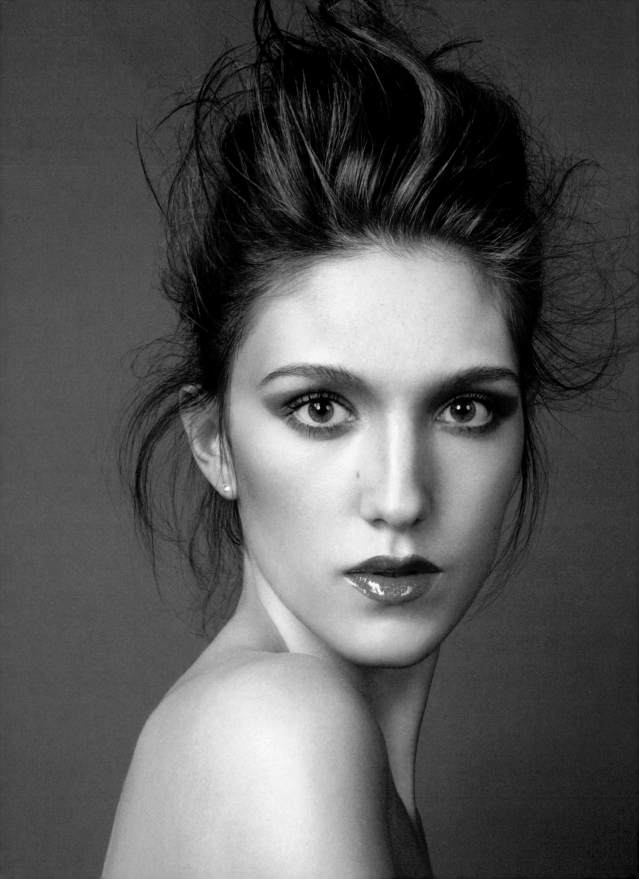

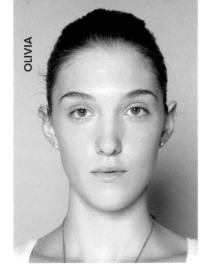
OLIVIA

The most important tool for this look is concealer. When you have used graphic shapes and straight edges, use concealer to sharpen the lip outline and eyeshadow edges afterwards.

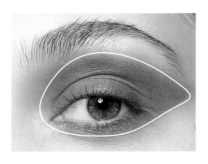

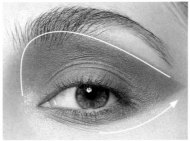

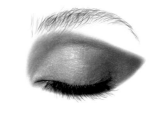

1. EYESHADOW
Circle your eye with brown eyeshadow. Extend the eyeshadow well beyond the outer corner of the eye and finish in a point.

2. SHARPEN
Apply the eyeshadow all the way up to the brow line. Put some concealer on a brush and use it to sharpen the eyeshadow point.

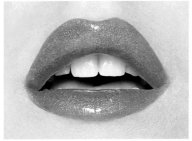

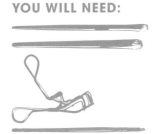

3. MASCARA
Use an eyelash curler for that perfect eyelash sweep. Then apply mascara thoroughly to the lashes, not forgetting the hairs at the inner and outer corners of the eye.

4. LIPSTICK & GLOSS
Apply a vibrant pink lipstick using a lip brush. Coat the lips with a clear gloss. Apply concealer to the corners of the mouth to sharpen the outline.

YOU WILL NEED:

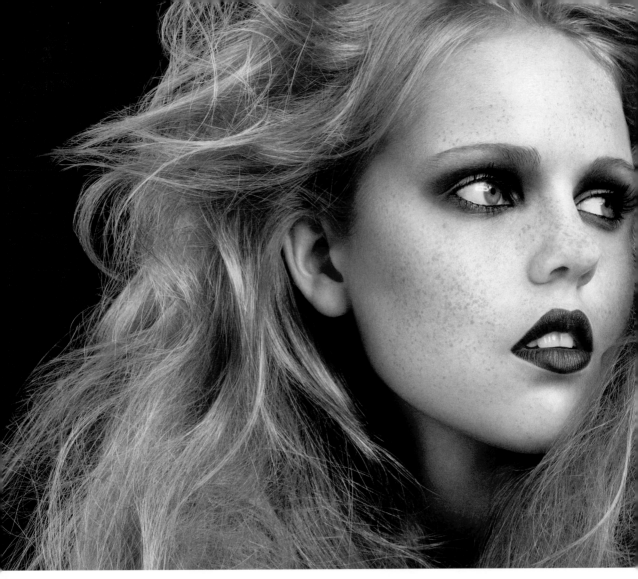

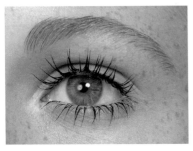

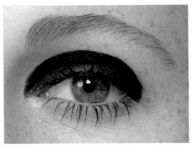

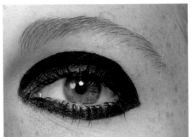

1. EYELASHES

Use an eyelash curler to shape your eyelashes before applying mascara. Apply several layers of mascara along the lash line and then apply it to the tips of the lashes.

2. PENCIL EYELINER

Starting from the outer corner of the eye, apply soft black pencil eyeliner over the entire mobile lid. The highest point should lie directly above the pupil.

3. CIRCLE

For smokey eyes, it is important that the colour encircles the entire eye. Only apply a little bit of pencil eyeliner beneath the lower lash line.

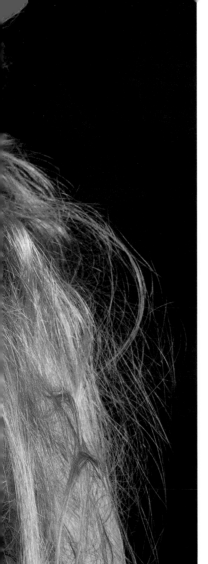

BASIC TECHNIQUES: SMOKEY EYES

To create smokey eyes, you need a good mastery of technique. By following these six steps, you will easily be able to create this look for yourself.

/**TIP:** Smokey eyes are extremely sexy not just in classic black, but also in muted colours such as dark blue, grey, or brown. Don't be unnerved: the first steps often look extreme. When this technique is combined with intensity, the result is an utterly sensational look.

YOU WILL NEED:

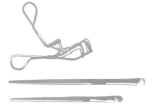

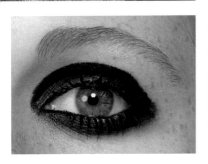

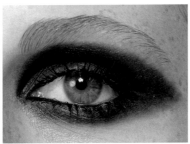

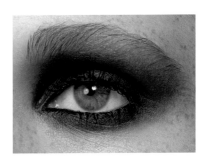

4. INTENSIFY

Applying pencil eyeliner to the inner rim of the eye gives the eye a dramatic look. Line the inside corner of the eye, too, which makes the white of the eye look even whiter.

5. SHADOW

Set the eyeliner with eyeshadow, and taper it out over the edge of the eyeliner to the outside corner of the eye so there are no hard edges.

6. BLEND

Using a clean brush, blend in the edges of the eyeshadow up and into the brow line.

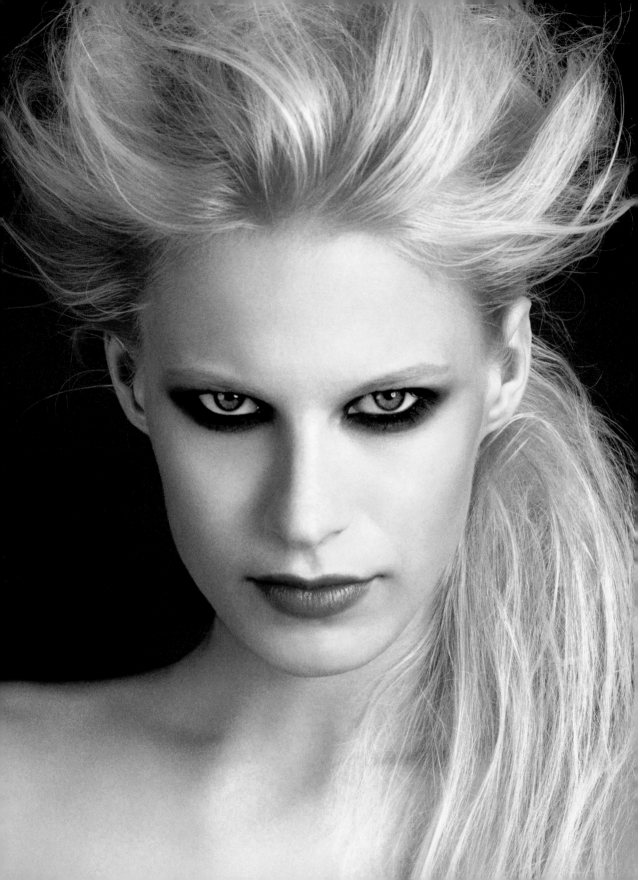

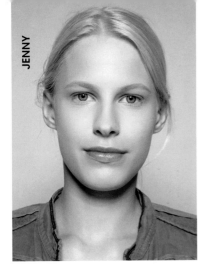

JENNY

Pencil eyeliner is the base for smokey eyes. The eyeliner has to be soft and oily, otherwise this technique will not succeed.

/TIP: If you are using intense colours, you can do your make-up in reverse order. Make up your eyes first, then correct any little mistakes. When the eye make-up is finished, apply concealer and foundation to your face as usual.

YOU WILL NEED:

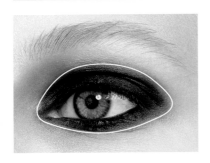

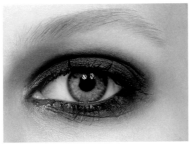

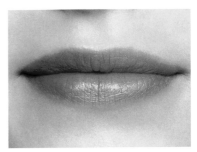

1. PENCIL EYELINER & EYESHADOW

Circle the entire eye with black pencil eyeliner. Then cover the liner with chocolate brown eyeshadow to fix it and gently blend it in.

2. MASCARA

Apply mascara to the lashes, starting as close to the lash line as possible. Take your time to ensure no mascara lands on the eyeshadow.

3. LIPSTICK

Use a skin-coloured lip liner to trace the lip line. This makes the lips look more even. Dab on silky, matte lipstick with a fingertip.

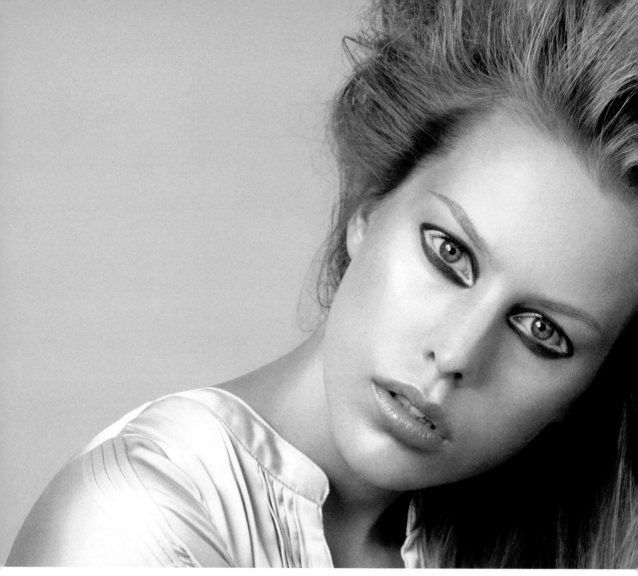

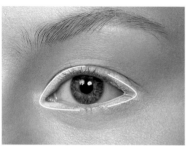

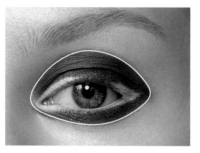

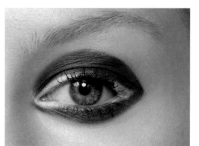

1. WHITE PENCIL EYELINER

Apply white pencil eyeliner to the inner and outer corners of the eyes in the shape of a "v". Be careful not to allow the two lines to meet above or below the pupil.

2. EYESHADOW

Using a small brush, circle the eye with blue eyeshadow. Take care not to cover the white pencil eyeliner. Tidy up the edges with a cotton bud.

3. MASCARA

Curl your eyelashes and apply thick layers of mascara above and below the pupil. Place a spoon along the upper lash line to avoid getting mascara on the eyeshadow.

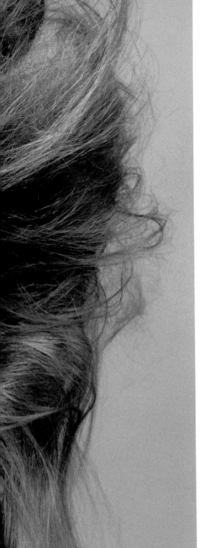

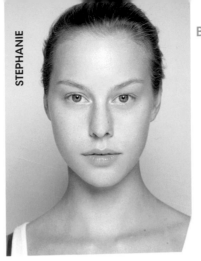

STEPHANIE

/**TIP:** The most important thing to think about when using eyeshadow is how you want it to end at the outer corner of the eye. You can choose between pointed, angled, or blended-in and completely change the look. Just alter the style to your liking.

YOU WILL NEED:

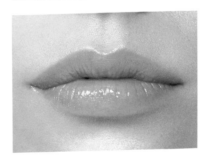

4. **BLUSHER**
Apply blusher to the cheekbone and blend it in upwards, downwards, and on the sides.

5. **GLOSS**
Finally, apply a lightly tinted gloss to the lips, working evenly from the outside to the centre of the mouth.

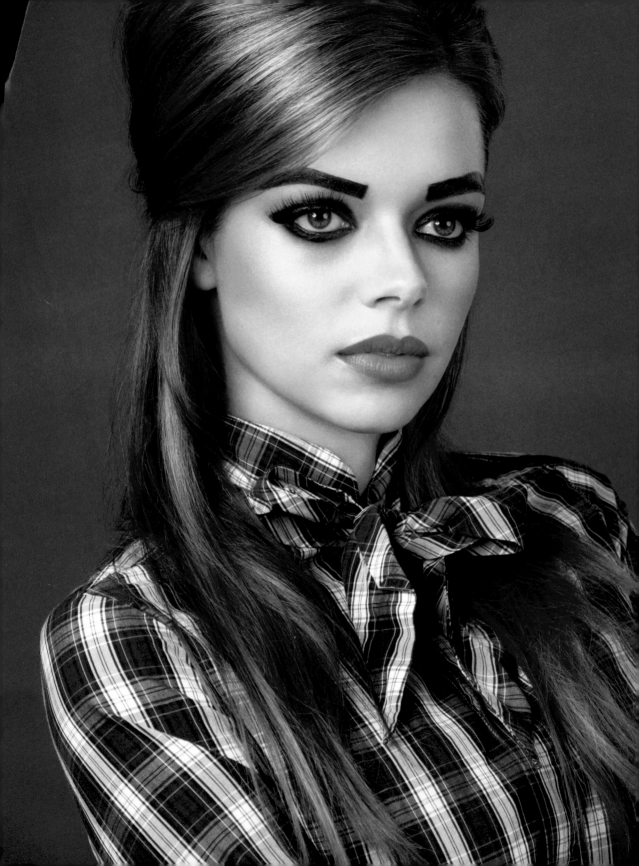

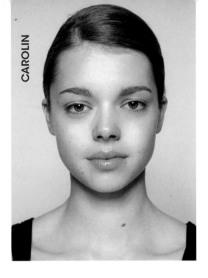

CAROLIN

For this extreme look, lipstick in a delicate shade of reddish-brown is the best choice so that the eyes remain the focal point.

/**TIP:** This look pairs trendy eyebrows with highly accented eyes. If the pitch-black pencil eyeliner used for this look is too adventurous for you, you can also use a dark brown colour – just experiment a bit. To finish off this extravagant eyebrow look, reddish-brown lipstick is just the thing.

YOU WILL NEED:

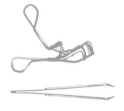

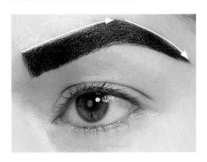

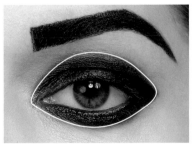

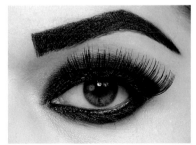

1. EYEBROWS

This is really easy to do. Start the line above the inner corner of the eye. Then take the line upwards for two-thirds of the length, and downwards for one-third. End the eyebrow higher than its starting point.

2. PENCIL EYELINER

Using soft black pencil eyeliner, outline the entire eye including the inner rim. Tidy up the lines with a cotton bud.

3. EXTRA-LONG EYELASHES

Everything is extreme about this look. This is why false eyelashes are used. You can learn how to apply fake eyelashes perfectly on page 82.

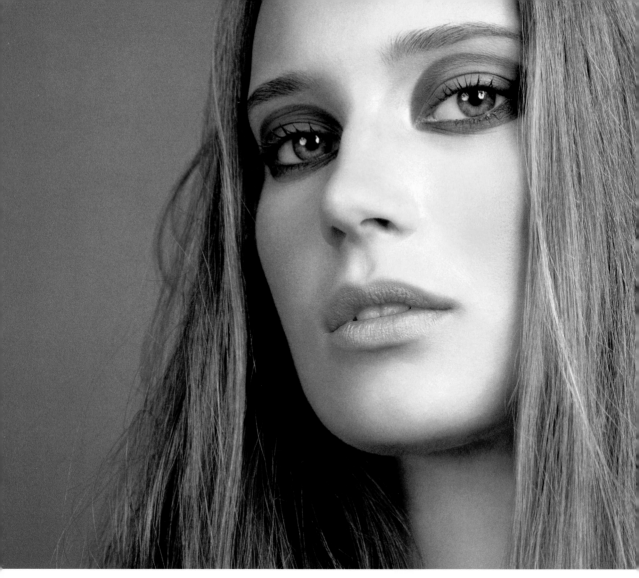

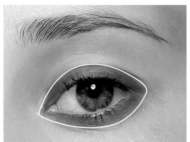

1. BASE COLOUR
Circle the eye evenly in an almond-shape using a saturated orange colour. To make a well-defined outline, use a brush with short, thick bristles.

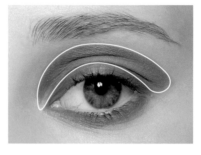

2. SECOND COLOUR
Evenly apply the second eyeshadow over the top edge of the orange shadow up into the eye crease. For deeper colour intensity, use a brush with short, thick bristles.

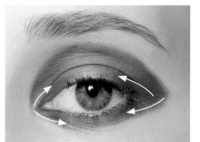

3. SHADING
Brush more of the second colour over the orange eyeshadow on the upper and lower lids from both corners of the eye to the centre. This closes up the eyeshadow.

MARIE-THERESE

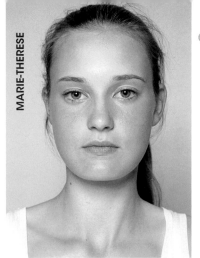

/**TIP:** To make the eyes look bigger, apply eye make-up to the inner and outer corners of the eyes. Close up the eyeshadow so the upper and lower eyeshadows meet. The eyeshadow must be continous. Always begin applying eyeshadow at the inner corner of the eye, otherwise the eye will be shortened visually.

YOU WILL NEED:

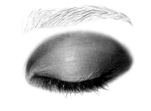

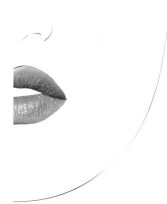

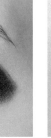
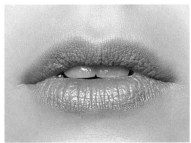

4. MASCARA & PENCIL EYELINER

Apply mascara thickly to the upper and lower lashes. Using blue pencil eyeliner on the lower inner rim brings your own eye colour to the fore, as the contrast is higher.

5. LIPS

With such strong eye make-up the lips should be understated. Here, a little lip balm is used, then shimmery eyeshadow is dabbed on the lips.

47 \ SHOW GIRL

YOU WILL NEED:

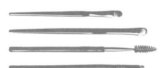

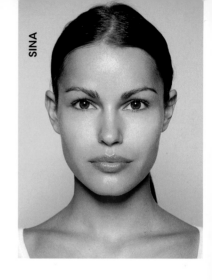

SINA

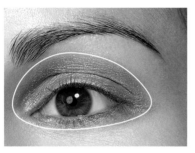

1. CIRCLE
Circle the entire eye in an almond shape with shimmery-blue eyeshadow.

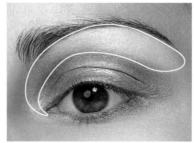

2. HIGHLIGHT
Start applying the lighter eyeshadow at the inner corner of the eye, blending it up to the brow line.

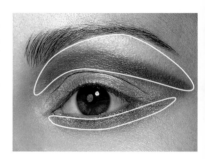

3. EYESHADOW
A third colour, a lilac shade, is brushed below the brow and into the eye crease. Also apply eyeshadow along the lower lash line.

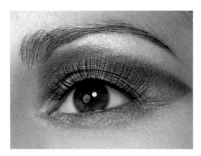

4. MASCARA
Brush the eyebrows to remove any loose powder and apply mascara along the lash line. Then apply mascara to the tips of the lashes.

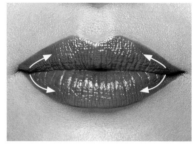

5. LIPSTICK
The easiest way to outline lips is to use a lip brush, always work from the outer corners to the centre. Once the outline is complete, fill in the rest of your lips using the lip brush.

/TIP: You don't need a lip liner to create the perfect lip line. For this look, only a lip brush and lipstick were used. Put a lot of lipstick on your brush and run it right along the contour of your lips. The extra colour on the brush makes it easy to draw a perfect outline.

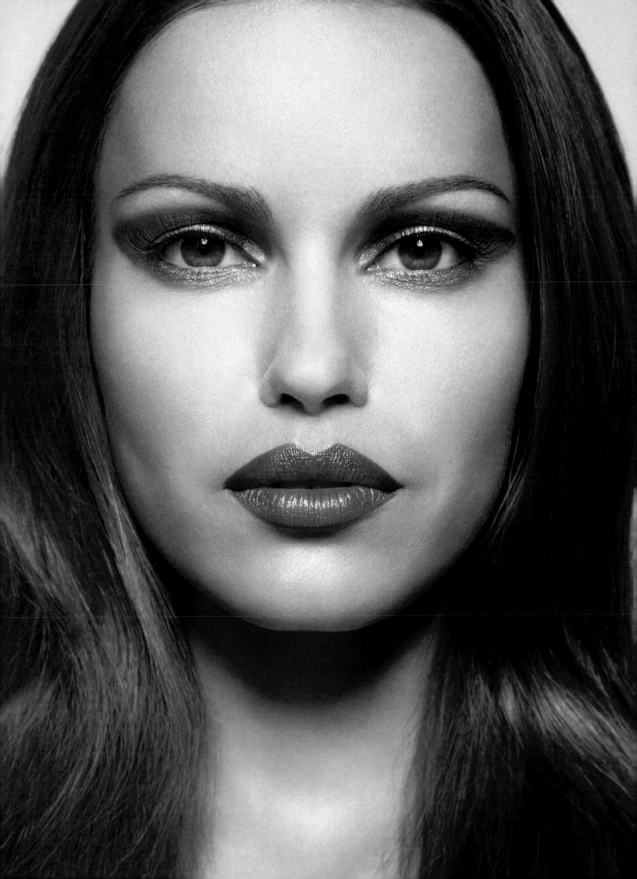

JUMI

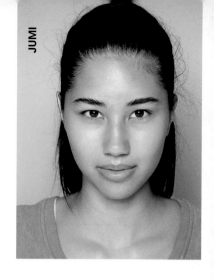

YOU WILL NEED:

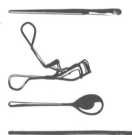

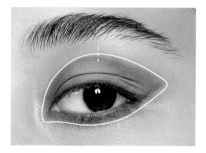

1. EYESHADOW
Circle your eye with eyeshadow in an almond shape. The highest point should lie above the pupil.

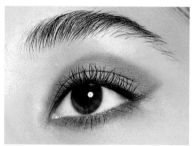

2. MASCARA
Curl your eyelashes with an eyelash curler first. To avoid getting mascara on the eyeshadow, place a spoon along the upper lash line and apply the mascara over the spoon.

/TIP: No matter what shape of eyes you have, when applying eyeshadow in an almond shape, take care that the tip of the eyeshadow extends beyond the outer corner of the eye. Otherwise the lid will appear droopy.

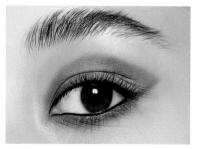

3. PENCIL EYELINER
To emphasize almond-shaped eyes more intensely, use black pencil eyeliner. Draw an even line on the inner corner of the eye.

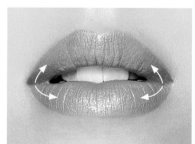

4. LIPSTICK
A shimmery pink colour makes a great contrast to the rich green. Apply the lipstick with a brush and always work from the corners of the lips to the centre.

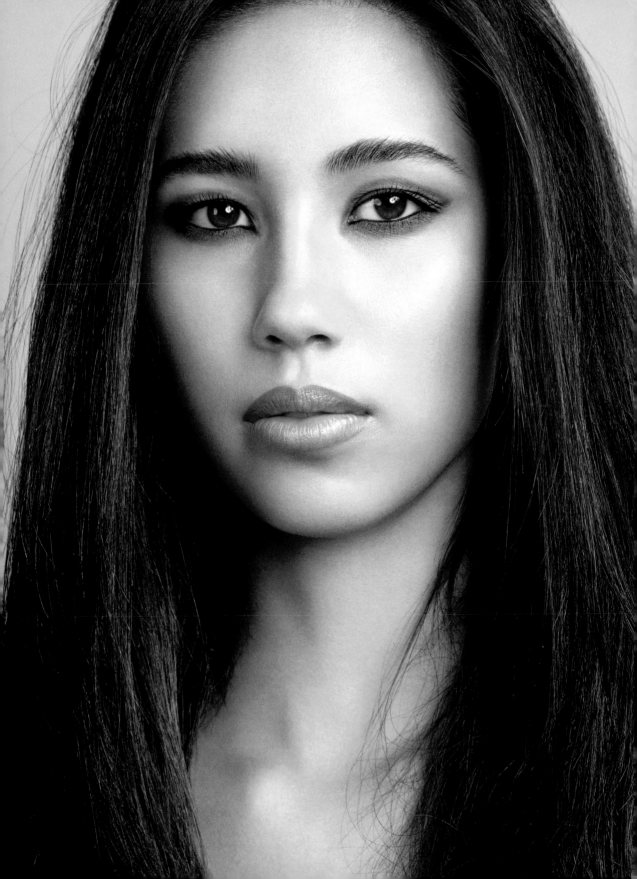

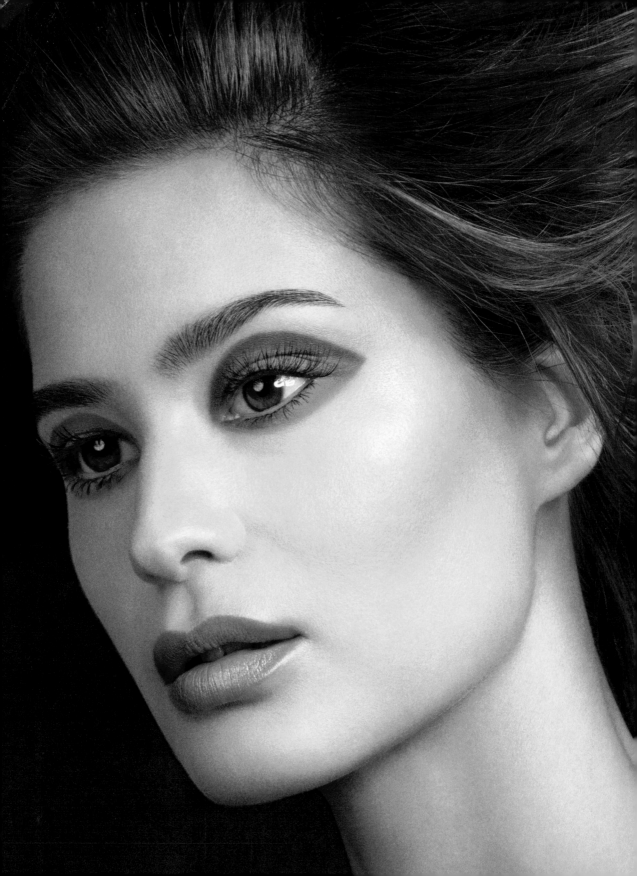

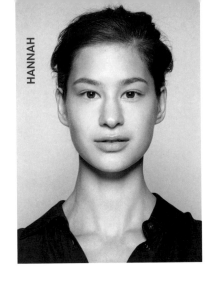

Here, two intense colours are used to create a highly dramatic look. You can also create a great look with subtler colours.

/TIP: This look, with its extra-strong colours, shows you how much can be done with graphic shapes. This make-up style also demonstrates how hooded eyes can be disguised just by using two colours. With your eye open, draw an arch on your upper eyelid. Choose colours that appeal to you and suit your mood. For hooded eyes, just make sure to apply the deeper shade above the eye crease.

YOU WILL NEED:

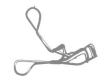

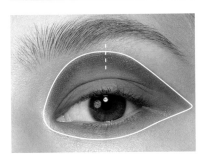

1. EYESHADOW
Circle the open eye with pink eyeshadow in an almond shape. The highest point should lie above the pupil. Draw the upper arch with lilac eyeshadow.

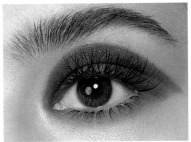

2. EYELASHES
Curl the eyelashes with an eyelash curler and apply masara thickly to the upper and lower lashes.

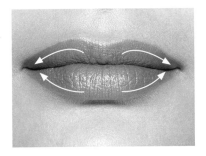

3. LIPS
Apply shiny lipstick to the centre of the lips and smooth it out to the sides.

BASIC TECHNIQUES: EYEBROWS

Using mascara on the brows emphasizes the eyes and looks very natural. Eyeshadow and pencil eyeliner sculpt the eyebrows wonderfully.

/MASCARA

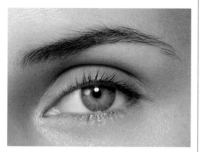

1. LOWEST POINT
Eyebrow mascara is great for quickly emphasizing the brow in a natural-looking way. Begin at the lowest point.

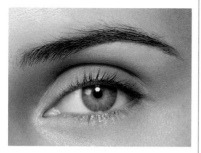

2. BROW MASCARA
Wipe the wand on a cloth. There still will be enough mascara on the wand to define the brow and yet keep it natural-looking. Using long strokes, brush the eyebrow hairs in the direction of hair growth.

/EYESHADOW

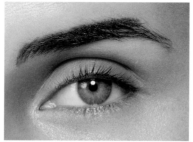

1. HIGHEST POINT
To fill in the eyebrow and emphasize the brow arch, use eyebrow powder or matte eyeshadow.

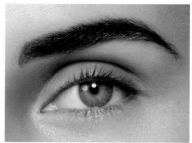

2. FILL-IN
Draw very fine lines in the direction of hair growth with eyeshadow, and then use a small brush to blend in the lines.

/EYEBROW PENCIL

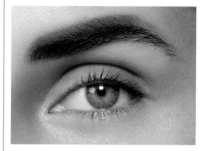

1. HIGHEST POINT
Use pencil eyeliner to fill in any gaps. The highest point of the eyebrow should lie above the outer corner of the eye.

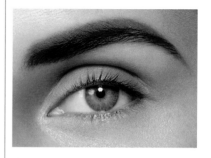

2. FILL-IN
Use an eyebrow pencil to pencil-in fine lines that follow the shape of the eyebrow. Draw in the direction of hair growth. Then brush the brow with an eyebrow brush.

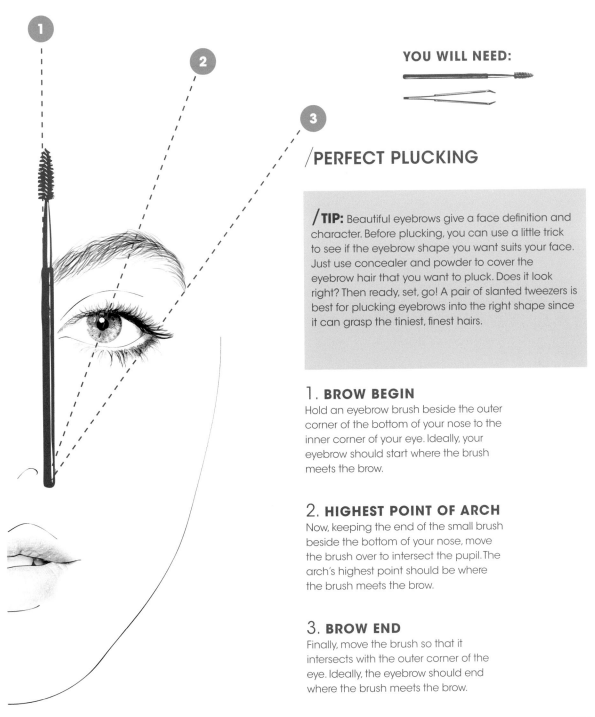

/PERFECT PLUCKING

/**TIP:** Beautiful eyebrows give a face definition and character. Before plucking, you can use a little trick to see if the eyebrow shape you want suits your face. Just use concealer and powder to cover the eyebrow hair that you want to pluck. Does it look right? Then ready, set, go! A pair of slanted tweezers is best for plucking eyebrows into the right shape since it can grasp the tiniest, finest hairs.

1. BROW BEGIN

Hold an eyebrow brush beside the outer corner of the bottom of your nose to the inner corner of your eye. Ideally, your eyebrow should start where the brush meets the brow.

2. HIGHEST POINT OF ARCH

Now, keeping the end of the small brush beside the bottom of your nose, move the brush over to intersect the pupil. The arch's highest point should be where the brush meets the brow.

3. BROW END

Finally, move the brush so that it intersects with the outer corner of the eye. Ideally, the eyebrow should end where the brush meets the brow.

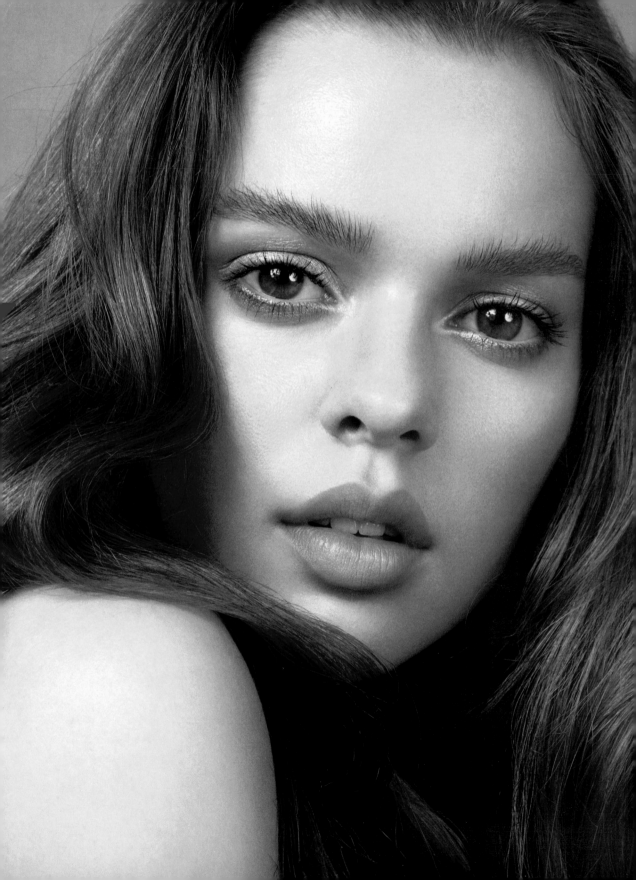

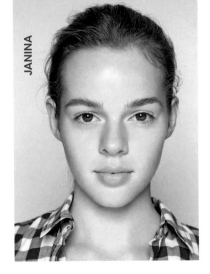

JANINA

Eyebrows are trendy! Using an eyebrow brush, or a toothbrush, brush the hairs upwards in the direction of hair growth. To make them stay in place, put some hairspray or gel on the brush.

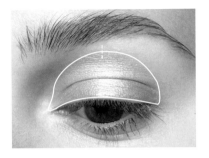

1. EYESHADOW

Apply apple-green eyeshadow over the upper lid using a large, rounded brush. The highest point should lie above the pupil. When the eye is open, the green should be just visible.

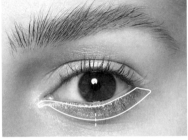

2. ACCENTS

Using an angled brush, apply delicate violet eyeshadow to accent the lower lash line. The lowest point should lie under the pupil, and the two colours should meet at the inner and outer corners of the eye.

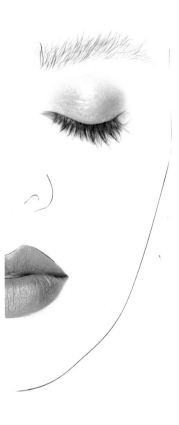

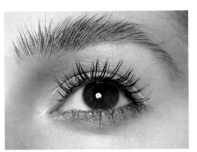

3. EYELASHES & EYEBROWS

Apply mascara, making sure to apply it more thickly to the bottom of the lashes than to the tips. Using an eyebrow brush, gently brush the eyebrows upwards.

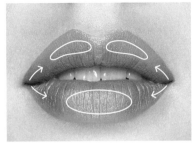

4. LIPSTICK

For a lovely outline, always work from the outside of the mouth to the centre. To finish, dab a bit of extra colour on the lips with a fingertip to draw attention to the centre of the lips.

YOU WILL NEED:

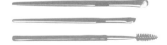

BEAUTY TIPS FOR EVERY AGE

You don't have to be twenty to experiment with make-up and try out new trends, colours, and textures. Whatever your age, there are certain things to watch out for.

/20+

When you are in your twenties, you can follow every trend, from extravagant runway looks to very pure, nude looks. The complexion usually is flawless and a perfect canvas for many make-up styles. Experiment to discover the colours that suit you best. **When in your twenties, concealer, blusher, and mascara are all you need to make you look fabulous! Eyeliner looks absolutely great too**, since it is easy to draw an exact line on smooth skin.

Youthful skin needs, if it needs anything at all, **very little foundation**. In this age group, those who use **moisturising cream with sun factor protection**, will protect their skin for decades to come.

Usually it is enough to apply **concealer to blemishes or to make small skin discolorations disappear** – the skin instantly looks flawless. At the most, use a light foundation.

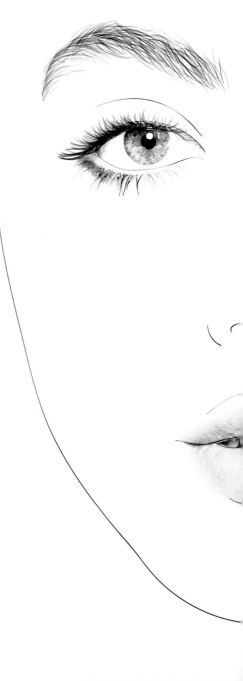

/30+

By thirty, you have discovered your personal style; it just needs to be perfected. Small tricks help you look fresher and more alert. Also, you still should be adventurous enough to play with current trends that showcase your own personality. Whatever you do, avoid using muted and subtle colours.

Foundation becomes more important at thirty, since it covers up redness and tired skin perfectly, and your skin looks smoother when you use it. **Make sure to choose two shades of foundation.** This lets you blend two colours together to create the skin tone and contours ideal for you. Products you should always have on hand are **concealer for shadows around your eyes, and eyeshadow in complementary colours** to make the eyes glow.

The way you apply mascara and foundation is now routine, but it isn't quite perfect. **When you are applying mascara, make sure to apply mascara to the fine hairs at the inner and outer corners of the eye.** Foundation should always look natural and seem to meld with the skin so make sure to blend it in well so no edges can be seen.

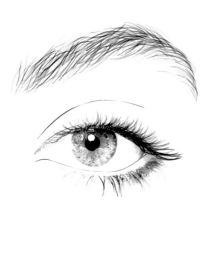

/40+

What looked good during the past twenty years might no longer be right for you today. Using an eye cream to reduce the first signs of wrinkles, and visiting a beautician, will help you to keep looking vibrant. **Expression lines are great, since they reflect character and personality.**

Applying liquid eyeliner accurately becomes more difficult, because the skin around the eyes is less elastic. Just apply eyeliner along the lash line and forget about fancy eyeliner flips. **Always use an eyelash curler to help enhance the eyes.**

The idea that women over forty should have shorter hair and only wear discreet make-up is completely outdated. **It is important to use make-up that covers well**, this is especially important for foundation. Only apply a thin coat of foundation so that the complexion looks natural. **Also, only use concealer to cover up shadows**, otherwise attention will be drawn to any wrinkles. **Choose intense colours of eyeshadow and lipstick** for a fabulous effect.

/50+

If you are in your fifties, you know very well what pleases you and how to create a desired effect. However, skin does change. The rule of thumb is **the more mobile your face, the softer your make-up should be.** Liquid eyeliner only serves to give more emphasis to the laughter lines around the eye, and a sharp lip line brings small skin creases to the fore.

The best tactic is to **focus attention on the area around the eyes.** This is done by selecting a **dark eyeshadow colour**, that is then softened. **Only use foundation sparingly** so that nothing lodges in the creases. **Mascara and an eyelash curler are an absolute must for luminous, alert eyes.** Applying blusher makes the skin look very even and the face well defined.

Be careful when choosing shades of blusher – **pick vibrant, soft colours.** A great way of making your skin look vibrant is to use a **hint of bronzing powder.** Choose intense to soft shades for your lips, but **avoid using glitter.** Lip gloss is easy to use and makes the lips look firmer and fuller.

S.O.S. TIPS

Tiny blemishes, chapped lips, and tired eyes? Don't panic! With the help of these handy tips, calamity will be averted in no time.

/TIP: To be prepared for any eventuality, always carry the following items in your make-up bag: a mirror; concealer, for quickly making yourself look fresh; powder, for fighting shiny skin; cotton buds for fixing little mistakes; lipstick or lip gloss; and eyeshadow, for touching up your eye make-up.

/DARK CIRCLES

If you always have dark circles under your eyes, visit your dermatologist to explore possible causes and treatments. It might also help to cut down on sugar, white wheat flour, fruit juices, and soft drinks. Drinking two to three litres of water a day is beneficial, as it activates the metabolism and makes rings under the eyes disappear. When nothing else helps, reach for concealer and cover up small shadows.

/TIRED EYES

An eyelash curler is the best weapon to combat tired eyes. When you've given your eyelashes a nice upwards lift, just apply mascara along the upper lash line and colour your eyebrows with an eyebrow pencil. This will give more definition and a sharpness to your eye. To look even more alert, highlight the inner corner of each eye with pale eyeshadow and put a bit just under the eyebrows, too.

/SWOLLEN EYES

Cooling the eyes is the best thing to do when they are swollen. Place either a cooling eye mask or cold spoon on the eyes. Or brew chamomile tea, which has calming and anti-inflammatory properties, let the tea bags cool, and place a tea bag on each eye. This will give immediate relief. Only apply eye creams designed to reduce puffiness once the swelling has died down.

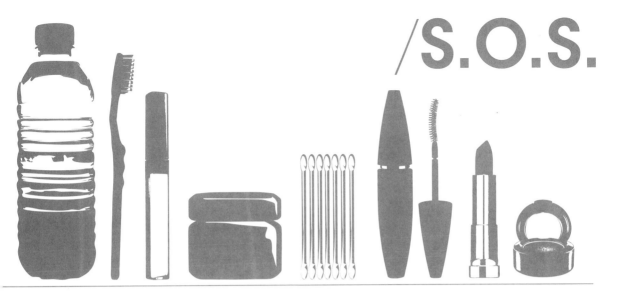

/BLEMISHES

The most important thing to remember about blemishes is to keep your hands away from your face and never to squeeze the blemishes, which just makes everything worse. If you suffer badly from blemishes, change your pillowcase several times a week and regularly disinfect anything that comes into contact with your hands and face. This doesn't just mean brushes and sponges, but also your mobile phone. If you want to cover up blemishes, first apply foundation as usual, and then use concealer to touch up where needed.

/DRY SKIN

If you have dry skin, it isn't enough to moisturise it; you also need to pay attention to your diet. Healthy skin isn't too dry or too oily. If you drink two to three litres of water a day, your skin's moisture balance will be restored and your skin will regenerate itself. Products containing natural substances are best if you have dry skin, since they are gentle on the skin and restore balance.

/OILY SKIN

Oily skin can develop for many reasons, such as using too many skincare products or a moisturiser that is much too rich. To help fight oily skin, cleanse your face just once, at night, and use a moisturiser that is optimal for your skin type. Sometimes it helps to take a brief break from using foundation so that the skin has a chance to recover. All other cosmetics, such as mascara and concealer, can be used without problems during a make-up break.

/SMUDGED MASCARA AND EYELINER

When mascara smears, it is often a sign that it is too old. Little smudges can best be removed with cotton buds. Pencil eyeliner tends to smudge much more often. Waterproof pencil eyeliner is the best choice, since it doesn't smudge. Avoid using oily eye cream before applying eye make-up since the make-up won't last as long. There are new cream pencil eyeliners on the market that turn powdery after application.

/CHAPPED LIPS

Chapped lips also are often caused by a lack of hydration or by applying too much lip balm. Regularly brushing the surface of your lips with a toothbrush, which is effectively a mini-exfoliation, increases the blood flow to the lips and prevents dead skin cells from even forming. A good method of treating chapped lips is to apply honey to them at night. This makes the lips especially soft.

/BROKEN CAPILLIARIES

Foundation generally doesn't provide enough cover to make broken capilliaries disappear. But, by using a concealer that is the same shade as your skin, you will be able to cover up any redness perfectly. Simply dab it on and pat it gently into the skin. Then apply foundation as usual.

/BORIS ENTRUP

Boris Entrup began his career in the classic way by training as a hair stylist. He then became an international assistant to many well-known and acclaimed hair- and make-up artists before becoming independent and launching his stellar career. Boris has been the exclusive make-up artist for Maybelline Jade since 2007. At the same time, he has continued working as a make-up artist and beauty expert for countless international companies, and on photo shoots, television productions, fashion shows, and magazines. His clients are not only models working in the fashion and beauty industry, but also well-known personalities who use his talents when they make public appearances. The ideas of this passionate, creative, make-up artist influence modern trends. Boris also translates international runway looks for daily use.

/BILLIE SCHEEPERS

Born in Berlin, Billie Scheepers studied photography in Munich between 1999 and 2003. She then moved to London, where she still is based today. Billie assisted many international photographers, such as David Slijper and Nick Knight. Since 2006, she has been an independent photographer specialising in beauty, portrait, and fashion photography. Her work is inspired by paintings and sculptures of the Old Masters. Fittingly, her trademark is bringing traditional and classic techniques and themes into the present day. She combines technical precision with a female aesthetic and visual language.

/ACKNOWLEDGMENTS

My first thank you goes to the tremendous team that came together to create this book and helped me realise my idea in such a constructive and creative way. A big thank you to Billie Sheepers, first and foremost, who accurately reflected my ideas with her visual imagery. Thank you to Michael Schmidt, who patiently worked as my hair and make-up assistant over the course of the entire production, and to Yasmina Foudhaili, who never lost her nerve, although she got married while the book was being produced.

I would like to thank Monika Schlitzer of Dorling Kindersley Verlag for such loving realisation of my idea, and TELLUS Publishing, for their enthusiastic and creative collaboration. Here, special thanks go to Marie-Therese Kunth for project management and Jennifer Stoppel for layout and illustration.

Special thanks also to the model agencies 4play Modelmanagement, AWA Models International, Body & Soul Modelagentur, Louisa Models, md management, Mega Model Agency, MODEL MANAGEMENT, model team, Modelwerk, MUGA Modelmanagement, place models, Promod Model Agency, and all the models who featured in this book.

Lastly, I would like to thank my manager, Sigrid Engelniederhammer (BrandFaktor) who, as usual, considerately and unwaveringly steered me throughout the entire project. Thank you, Jens Puppe, for the links that you made!

/MODEL-AGENCIES

4play Modelmanagement
Gasstr. 4
D-22761 Hamburg
Tel. +49 40 87 97 62 92
www.4playhamburg.de
Models: Imke, Leandra, Nele,
Sarah, Sina, Stephanie

AWA Models International
Böttgerstr. 13
D-20148 Hamburg
Tel. +49 40 94 79 24 33
www.awa-models.de
Models: Akvile, Carolin

Body&Soul Modelagentur
Isestr. 23
D-20144 Hamburg
Tel. +49 40 41 20 91
www.bodyandsoul-models.de
Models: Charlotte, Joana,
Jessica

Louisa Models
Feldbrunnenstr. 24
D-20148 Hamburg
Tel. +49 40 414 40 - 100
www.louisa-models.de
Model: Laura

md management
Eppendorfer Weg 213
D-20253 Hamburg
Tel. +49 40 421 07 66 60
www.md-management.com
Models: Julia, Kamille, Nell,
Olivia, Romy

Mega Model Agency – Hamburg
Kaiser-Wilhelm-Str. 93
D-20355 Hamburg
Tel. +49 40 355 22 00
www.megamodel.de
Model: Marie-Therese

MODEL MANAGEMENT
Heidi Gross GmbH & Co. KG
Hartungstr. 5
D-20146 Hamburg
Tel. +49 40 44 05 55
www.model-management.de
Models: Carlotta, Georgia, Patricia

model team
Schlüterstr. 60
D-20146 Hamburg
Tel. +49 40 41 41 03 - 0
www.modelteam-hamburg.de
Models: Janina, Kangeh, Lena

Modelwerk
Modelagentur GmbH
Rothenbaumchaussee 1
D-20148 Hamburg
Tel. +49 40 88 30 73 - 0
www.modelwerk.de
Model: Sara (Look 33)

MUGA Modelmanagement
Studio 111
Langenfelder Str. 111
D-22769 Hamburg
Tel. +49 40 881 44 99 13
www.muga-model.de
Models: Michelle, Vivien

place models hamburg
Am Felde 29
D-22765 Hamburg
Tel. +49 40 460 79 60
www.placemodels.com
Models: Hannah, Jenny, Sara, Sarice

Promod Model Agency
Semoerstr. 32
D-22303 Hamburg
Tel. +49 40 471 00 00
www.promod.org
Models: Jumi, Lovelyn

/PHOTOGRAPHY EQUIPMENT

KNACKSCHARF GmbH & Co. KG
Grindelhof 48–50
20146 Hamburg
Tel. +49 40 33 60 33
www.knackscharf-rent.de

/BORIS ENTRUP'S MANAGEMENT

BrandFaktor
Die Markenmacher
Sigrid Engelniederhammer
Augsburgerstr. 12
80337 München
Tel. +49 89 202 31 94
www.brandfaktor.com

/COPYRIGHT

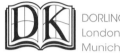
DORLING KINDERSLEY
London, New York, Melbourne,
Munich, Delhi

TELLUS CORPORATE MEDIA GMBH
PROJECT EDITOR Marie-Therese Kunth
DESIGNER Jennifer Stoppel
PHOTOGRAPHY Billie Scheepers Photography,
www.billiescheepers.com, also:
L'Oréal Deutschland GmbH for product photography pp 13, 20 & 21
CREATIVE TECHNICAL SUPPORT Adi Admoni, Dennis Bauermeister
ILLUSTRATION Jennifer Stoppel
HAIR & MAKE-UP Boris Entrup
HAIR & MAKE-UP ASSISTANCE Michael Schmidt
TEXT & PHOTO PRODUCTION Boris Entrup, www.borisentrup.com
EDITOR Yasmina Foudhaili
PROOFREADING Claudia Celentano, Lars Freitag
COLOUR REPRODUCTION ALPHABETA GmbH, Hamburg,
www.alphabeta.de

DK GERMANY
PUBLISHING DIRECTOR Monika Schlitzer
PRODUCTION DIRECTOR Dorothee Whittaker
SENIOR EDITOR Gabriele Kalmbach

DK LONDON
TRANSLATOR Barbara Hopkinson
PROJECT EDITOR Elizabeth Yeates
MANAGING EDITOR Dawn Henderson
MANAGING ART EDITOR Christine Keilty
EDITORIAL ASSISTANT Elizabeth Clinton
DESIGN ASSISTANT Kate Fenton
SENIOR PRODUCER, PRE-PRODUCTION Tony Phipps
SENIOR PRODUCER Alex Bell
ART DIRECTOR Peter Luff
PUBLISHER Peggy Vance

First published in Great Britain in 2014
by Dorling Kindersley Limited, 80 Strand, London WC2R 0RL
Penguin Group (UK)

Copyright © 2014 Dorling Kindersley Limited

1 2 3 4 5 6 7 8 9 10
001–196222–Apr/2014

A CIP catalogue record for this book is available from the British Library.

ISBN 978-1-4093-3806-2

Printed and bound by South China (DK)

Discover more at www.dk.com